Dermatology

Editor

KRISTEN M. GRIPPE

PHYSICIAN ASSISTANT CLINICS

www.physicianassistant.theclinics.com

Consulting Editor
JAMES A. VAN RHEE

April 2016 • Volume 1 • Number 2

ELSEVIER

1600 John F. Kennedy Boulevard ● Suite 1800 ● Philadelphia, Pennsylvania, 19103-2899

http://www.theclinics.com

PHYSICIAN ASSISTANT CLINICS Volume 1, Number 2
April 2016 ISSN 2405-7991, ISBN-13: 978-0-323-44363-0

Editor: Jessica McCool
Developmental Editor: Casey Jackson

Physician Assistant Clinics (ISSN: 2405–7991) is published quarterly by Elsevier Inc., 360 Park Avenue South, New York, NY 10010-1710. Months of issue are January, April, July, and October. Periodicals postage paid at New York, NY and additional mailing offices. Subscription prices are $150.00 per year (US individuals), $195.00 (US institutions), $100.00 (US students), $150.00 (Canadian individuals), $245.00 (Canadian institutions), $100.00 (Canadian students), $150.00 (international individuals), $245.00 (international institutions), and $100.00 (international students). Foreign air speed delivery is included in all *Clinics* subscription prices. All prices are subject to change without notice. POSTMASTER: Send address changes to *Physician Assistant Clinics*, Elsevier Periodicals Customer Service, 11830 Westline Industrial Drive, St. Louis, MO 63146. Customer Service Health Sciences Division, Subscription Customer Service, 3251 Riverport Lane, Maryland Heights, MO 63043. **Customer Service: 1-800-654-2452 (U.S. and Canada); 314-447-8871 (outside U.S. and Canada). Fax: 314-447-8029. E-mail: journalscustomerservice-usa@elsevier.com (for print support); journalsonlinesupport-usa@elsevier.com (for online support).**

Reprints. For copies of 100 or more, of articles in this publication, please contact the Commercial Reprints Department, Elsevier Inc., 360 Park Avenue South, New York, NY 10010-1710. Tel. 212-633-3874; Fax: 212-633-3820; E-mail: reprints@elsevier.com.

Physician Assistant Clinics is covered in *MEDLINE/PubMed (Index Medicus)* and *EMBASE/Excerpta Medica, Current Contents/Clinical Medicine, and ISI/BIOMED.*

PROGRAM OBJECTIVE
The goal of the *Physician Assistant Clinics* is to keep practicing physician assistants up to date with current clinical practice by providing timely articles reviewing the state of the art in patient care.

TARGET AUDIENCE
Physician Assistants and other healthcare professionals.

LEARNING OBJECTIVES
Upon completion of this activity, participants will be able to:
1. Review the diagnosis and management of melanoma and non-melanoma skin disorders.
2. Discuss the use of neurotoxins, dermal fillers, and topical therapies in dermatologic disorders.
3. Recognize clinical approaches to diffuse blisters and nail findings.

ACCREDITATION
The Elsevier Office of Continuing Medical Education (EOCME) is accredited by the Accreditation Council for Continuing Medical Education (ACCME) to provide continuing medical education for physicians.

The EOCME designates this enduring material for a maximum of 15 *AMA PRA Category 1 Credit*(s)™. Physicians should claim only the credit commensurate with the extent of their participation in the activity.

All other health care professionals requesting continuing education credit for this enduring material will be issued a certificate of participation.

DISCLOSURE OF CONFLICTS OF INTEREST
The EOCME assesses conflict of interest with its instructors, faculty, planners, and other individuals who are in a position to control the content of CME activities. All relevant conflicts of interest that are identified are thoroughly vetted by EOCME for fair balance, scientific objectivity, and patient care recommendations. EOCME is committed to providing its learners with CME activities that promote improvements or quality in healthcare and not a specific proprietary business or a commercial interest.

The planning committee, staff, authors and editors listed below have identified no financial relationships or relationships to products or devices they or their spouse/life partner have with commercial interest related to the content of this CME activity:
Heather Adams, MPAS, PA-C; Theodore Alkousakis, MD; Risha Bellomo, MPAS, PA-C; Renata M. Block, MMS, PA-C; Eileen Cheever, MPAS, PA-C; Jennifer Conner, MPAS, PA-C; Chelsey Coven, MPAS, PA-C; Joseph Daniel; Ramin Fathi, MD; Anjali Fortna; Kristen M. Grippe, MPAS, PA-C; Lewis Kevin Harrington, ARNP, FNP-C; Mark Hyde, MMS, PA-C; Casey Jackson; Tarannum Jaleel, MD; Jolene R. Jewell, MD; Young Kwak, MD; Jessica McCool; Sarah A. Myers, MD; Christie Riemer, BS; Naveed Sami, MD; Martha L. Sikes, MS, RPh, PA-C; Jonathan Soh, BS; Megan Suermann; Philip E. Tobin, DHSc, PA-C.

The planning committee, staff, authors and editors listed below have identified financial relationships or relationships to products or devices they or their spouse/life partner have with commercial interest related to the content of this CME activity:
James A. Van Rhee, MS, PA-C, DFAAPA receives royalties/patents from Kaplan, Inc.

UNAPPROVED/OFF-LABEL USE DISCLOSURE
The EOCME requires CME faculty to disclose to the participants:
1. When products or procedures being discussed are off-label, unlabelled, experimental, and/or investigational (not US Food and Drug Administration [FDA] approved); and
2. Any limitations on the information presented, such as data that are preliminary or that represent ongoing research, interim analyses, and/or unsupported opinions. Faculty may discuss information about pharmaceutical agents that is outside of FDA-approved labelling. This information is intended solely for CME and is not intended to promote off-label use of these medications. If you have any questions, contact the medical affairs department of the manufacturer for the most recent prescribing information.

TO ENROLL
The CME program is available to all Physician Assistant Clinics subscribers at no additional fee. To subscribe to the Physician Assistant Clinics, call customer service at 1-800-654-2452 or sign up online at www.physicianassistant.theclinics.com.

METHOD OF PARTICIPATION

In order to claim credit, participants must complete the following:

1. Complete enrolment as indicated above.
2. Read the activity.
3. Complete the CME Test and Evaluation. Participants must achieve a score of 70% on the test. All CME Tests and Evaluations must be completed online.

CME INQUIRIES/SPECIAL NEEDS

For all CME inquiries or special needs, please contact elsevierCME@elsevier.com.

Contributors

CONSULTING EDITOR

JAMES A. VAN RHEE, MS, PA-C, DFAAPA
Associate Professor, Program Director, Yale Physician Associate Program, Yale University, New Haven, Connecticut

EDITOR

KRISTEN M. GRIPPE, PA-C, MPAS
Assistant Professor, Physician Assistant Department, Gannon University, Erie, Pennsylvania; Distance CME Committee Co-Chair, Society of Dermatology Physician Assistants, Waterford, Pennsylvania

AUTHORS

HEATHER ADAMS, MPAS, PA-C
Assistant Professor, Gannon University, Erie, Pennsylvania

THEODORE ALKOUSAKIS, MD
Assistant Clinical Professor, Department of Dermatology, University of Colorado Denver, Aurora, Colorado

RISHA BELLOMO, MPAS, PA-C
Allele Medical, Orlando, Florida

RENATA M. BLOCK, MMS, PA-C, SDPA, ISDPA, AAPA, IAPA
Pinski Dermatology & Cosmetic Surgery, Chicago, Illinois

EILEEN CHEEVER, MPAS, PA-C
The Rockoff Dermatology Center, Andover, Massachusetts

JENNIFER CONNER, MPAS, PA-C
Sonterra Dermatology, San Antonio, Texas

CHELSEY COVEN, MPAS, PA-C
Cowansville, Pennsylvania

RAMIN FATHI, MD
Resident Physician, Department of Dermatology, University of Colorado Denver, Aurora, Colorado

KRISTEN M. GRIPPE, PA-C, MPAS
Assistant Professor, Physician Assistant Department, Gannon University, Erie, Pennsylvania; Distance CME Committee Co-Chair, Society of Dermatology Physician Assistants, Waterford, Pennsylvania

LEWIS KEVIN HARRINGTON, ARNP, FNP-C
Allele Medical, Orlando, Florida

MARK HYDE, MMS, PA-C
Huntsman Cancer Institute, The University of Utah, Salt Lake City, Utah

TARANNUM JALEEL, MD
Department of Dermatology, University of Alabama at Birmingham, Birmingham, Alabama

JOLENE R. JEWELL, MD
Chief Resident, Department of Dermatology, Duke University Medical Center, Durham, North Carolina

YOUNG KWAK, MD
Department of Dermatology, University of Alabama at Birmingham, Birmingham, Alabama

SARAH A. MYERS, MD
Associate Professor, Department of Dermatology, Duke University Medical Center, Durham, North Carolina

CHRISTIE RIEMER, BS
Department of Dermatology, Michigan State University College of Human Medicine, Grand Rapids, Michigan

NAVEED SAMI, MD
Associate Professor, Director, Autoimmune Bullous Disease Clinic, Department of Dermatology, University of Alabama at Birmingham, Birmingham, Alabama

MARTHA L. SIKES, MS, RPh, PA-C
Clinical Assistant Professor, Department of Physician Assistant Studies, Mercer University, Atlanta, Georgia

JONATHAN SOH, BS
Department of Dermatology, University of Rochester School of Medicine and Dentistry, Rochester, New York

PHILIP E. TOBIN, DHSc, PA-C
Clinical Assistant Professor, Department of Physician Assistant Studies, Mercer University, Atlanta, Georgia

Contents

The diagnosis and treatment of pigmented or melanocytic lesions is difficult and can be intimidating. This review gives a brief overview of melanocytic lesions, their origins, diagnosis, and treatment. Although there is not a clear screening consensus guideline, a discussion of current screening suggestions and evidence is included. Current staging and treatment guidelines for melanoma are reviewed.

There is a growing epidemic of nonmelanoma skin cancers in the United States. Precancerous growths occur in more than 58 million Americans. Left untreated, these can develop into the 2 most common nonmelanoma skin cancers: basal cell carcinoma and squamous cell carcinoma. With an estimated 3.5 million new cases of nonmelanoma skin cancers in 2012, and with 1 in every 5 Americans developing a skin cancer during their lifetime, the importance of patient education is arising outside the medical clinic from health care providers in dermatology clinics, who play a key role in prevention, early detection, and treatment.

Rosacea is a common, chronic dermatologic condition marked by several subtypes and varying degrees of severity. These factors can lead to difficult diagnosis, challenges in treatment, and disruption of quality of life. This article seeks to inform health care providers about the types of rosacea, psychosocial impacts of the diagnosis, importance of patient education, and available treatment options to optimize the care of patients who suffer with rosacea.

Cutis marmorata telangiectatica congenita (CMTC) is a rare congenital condition of unknown cause. It is characterized by a pattern of reticulate erythema, known as cutis marmorata, as well as phlebectasia, and telangiectasia. Unlike benign cutis marmorata, it does not resolve with warming. CMTC can be associated with extracutaneous findings, making physical examination a critical component of diagnosis. Subcriteria addressing the occurrence of macrocephaly as a common extracutaneous finding have been a topic of debate. Prognosis for patients with CMTC can vary, with routine multidisciplinary follow-up suggested within the first years of life to monitor for any new abnormalities.

Cutaneous biopsies can provide important information regarding the pathology, severity, and treatment of skin disease. Familiarity with different skin biopsy techniques, and the clinical indications for each type of biopsy, helps maximize disease detection and patient satisfaction. This article provides a comprehensive overview of the indications for skin biopsy, various biopsy and suture techniques, wound care, and complications. This article outlines methodologies for the most common biopsy techniques used in dermatologic practice: curettage, snip, shave, saucerization, punch/core biopsy, and incisional and excisional in toto.

Topical medications are the foundation upon which dermatologic care is built. The proper use of topical therapeutics requires consideration of the active ingredient, potency, vehicle, and medication quantity. This article provides a concise but non-comprehensive list of topical medications used for acne, rosacea, psoriasis, actinic keratoses, and non-melanoma skin cancers. Common treatment regimens and pitfalls in prescribing topicals are discussed via clinical vignettes.

Some blistering eruptions are self-limited, but others are life threatening, and prompt diagnosis and management are critical. The clinical presentation of vesicles and bullae suggests a broad differential and this article (1) highlights some common diagnoses that may be encountered by primary care physicians and subspecialists, (2) provides a possible systematic diagnostic approach to such patients, including history, physical examination, and relevant work-up.

With the growing number of neurotoxin and dermal filler choices on the market for aesthetic enhancement it can be a cumbersome process to decide on what product is best for the patient. Having a clear understanding of the available products, product composition, longevity, mechanism of action, safety, shelf life, and product cost is crucial to the education of aesthetic patients on what product best suits their aesthetic needs and ultimately gives them the most natural and superior outcomes for which they are looking.

Examination of the nails can provide clues in determining systemic disorders before systemic manifestations signify underlying infection or even internal malignancy. Providers should be familiar with normal nail anatomy, specific history questions related to nail pathology, nail signs of systemic disease, and common nail findings. This review highlights normal nail anatomy, specific nail signs, and pertinent history, physical examination findings, and treatments of selected nail abnormalities.

Dermatology

PHYSICIAN ASSISTANT CLINICS

RELATED INTEREST

Medical Clinics of North America, November 2015 (Vol. 99, Issue 6)
Dermatology
Roy M. Colven, *Editor*
Available at: http://www.medical.theclinics.com/

THE CLINICS ARE AVAILABLE ONLINE!
Access your subscription at:
www.theclinics.com

Foreword

Dermatology

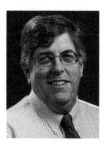

James A. Van Rhee, MS, PA-C, DFAAPA
Consulting Editor

According to the NCCPA (National Commission on Certification of Physician Assistants) 2014 Annual Report, currently 4.4% of all physician assistants work primarily in the specialty of dermatology.[1] Approximately 36% of all primary care office visits involve at least one skin problem, and for over half of these office visits, the skin problem is the chief compliant.[2] This issue of *Physician Assistant Clinics* is directed to the physician assistants outside of the dermatology specialty arena. But I am sure there is something for even the most experienced dermatology physician assistant in this issue.

Kristen Grippe, MPAS, PA-C, Assistant Professor at Gannon University Physician Assistant Program and a member of the Society of Dermatology Physician Assistants, is the guest editor for this issue, and she has selected a wide variety of topics and excellent authors. In this issue, we cover skin cancer from top to bottom. Hyde and Connor provide an excellent review of nevi to melanoma, and Block provides a review of nonmelanoma skin cancers. Need a review of biopsy and suture methodology? Then the article by Soh, Riemer, Alkousakis, and Fathi is for you. In that article, they cover the indications, contraindications, and methodology and provide a number of helpful suggestions for several of the common biopsy methods. Do you have questions about the wide variety of topical therapies? Then the article by Jewell and Myers will provide you with the answers as you work through a number of clinical scenarios in the article. Are stubborn nail infections a problem in your clinic? The article by Sikes and Tobin will provide you a variety of treatment options you can use in those tough situations.

I hope you enjoy the second issue of *Physician Assistant Clinics*. Our next issue will provide you with a review of Oncology.

Physician Assist Clin 1 (2016) xi–xii
http://dx.doi.org/10.1016/j.cpha.2016.01.002
2405-7991/16/$ – see front matter © 2016 Published by Elsevier Inc.

physicianassistant.theclinics.com

James A. Van Rhee, MS, PA-C, DFAAPA
Yale University
Yale Physician Associate Program
100 Church Street South, Suite A250
New Haven, CT 06519, USA

E-mail address:
james.vanrhee@yale.edu

REFERENCES

1. National Commission on Certification of Physician Assistants, Inc. March 2015. 2014 Statistical profile of certified physician assistants: an annual report of the National Commission on the Certification of Physician Assistants. Available at: http://www.nccpa.net/research.
2. Lowell BA, Froelich CW, Federman DG, et al. Dermatology in primary care: prevalence and patient disposition. J Am Acad Dermatol 2001;45(2):250–5.

Preface

Dermatology Is so Much More than "What Meets the Eye"

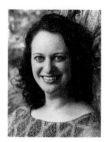

Kristen M. Grippe, PA-C, MPAS
Editor

With every patient encounter, physician assistants (PAs) have the opportunity to address dermatologic concerns. As the skin is the most visible organ, health care providers and patients alike have the ability to see when changes occur from either disease processes or chronologic aging, and patients are becoming more proactive in seeking advice from PAs about skin care. Unfortunately, the common perception that a suntan is "beautiful" has had several negative effects on long-term skin health due to prolonged sun bathing or tanning bed usage. Skin cancers are occurring more frequently and at younger ages, and self-esteem can be negatively impacted by chronic color changes and wrinkles. However, the specialty of dermatology is at an exciting time whereby research and knowledge are expanding in many positive ways. The field of cosmetic dermatology is quickly advancing to offer patients more effective treatment options for antiaging purposes, and new medications are currently available or on the horizon to treat a variety of skin diseases. After working in the field of dermatology for ten years, I have come to appreciate the amazing diversities of skin appearances. From children to the elderly, and with many different colors, there are endless variations that make every patient unique in their treatment desires and needs. The skin is also a very important organ with its crucial role in thermal regulation and protection from the external environment. The skin can also produce signs or symptoms that offer visible clues of many internal disease processes, sometimes before other symptoms are noticeable. As leaders in the health care field, PAs must be able to recognize an array of skin manifestations and guide our patients to make the best choices for skin health. I hope that this issue of *Physician Assistant Clinics* helps you to recognize the amazing qualities and importance of skin, so that you may realize that there is so much more to this diverse organ than what simply "meets the eye."

Physician Assist Clin 1 (2016) xiii–xiv
http://dx.doi.org/10.1016/j.cpha.2016.01.001
2405-7991/16/$ – see front matter © 2016 Published by Elsevier Inc.

physicianassistant.theclinics.com

Kristen M. Grippe, PA-C, MPAS
Gannon University
Physician Assistant Department
Erie, PA 16541, USA

Society of Dermatology Physician Assistants
8400 Westpark Dr. Fl 2
McLean, VA 22102, USA

E-mail address:
kgrippe@dermpa.org

From Nevi to Melanoma: Understanding the Basics of Lesions

 CrossMark

Mark Hyde, MMS, PA-C[a],*, Jennifer Conner, MPAS, PA-C[b]

KEYWORDS

- Melanoma • Nevus • Biopsy • Melanocyte origin

KEY POINTS

- PAs must understand the basic anatomic structure and cells that give rise to nevi and melanoma.
- It is important to know the main types of nevi and be able to identify them clinically.
- It is also important for PAs to know when and how to biopsy pigmented lesions and be able to identify the stage of melanoma and appropriate referral pattern based on the stage.

INTRODUCTION

Pigmented or melanocytic lesions are among the most commonly encountered skin lesions. These lesions span from simple lentigines, through nevi, into the realms of melanoma. Melanocyte origins and function are important to understand when evaluating or treating melanocytic lesions. One of the constant dilemmas facing clinicians is whether these lesions need to be biopsied or can be observed safely. Many different methods are in use as an aid to making this decision.

In this review of lesions of melanocytic origin, we discuss the embryologic roots of the melanocyte and the different lesions that originate from the melanocyte. In the course of this review on the melanocyte, clinical methods of determining atypia and deciding to biopsy or not will be explored. Finally, we outline the currently practiced literature supported methods of treating these entities. To accomplish this, we divide the discussion into the following 3 sections:

1. Melanocyte origin
2. Nevi
3. Melanoma

Disclosures: None.
[a] Huntsman Cancer Institute, The University of Utah, 2000 Circle of Hope, Suite 2281, Salt Lake City, UT 84112, USA; [b] Sonterra Dermatology, 325 E Sonterra Blvd #110, San Antonio, TX 78258, USA
* Corresponding author.
E-mail address: Mark.hyde@hci.utah.edu

Physician Assist Clin 1 (2016) 221–231
http://dx.doi.org/10.1016/j.cpha.2015.12.001
physicianassistant.theclinics.com

MELANOCYTE ORIGIN

The origin of the melanocyte is in the neural crest tissue of the human embryo. Melanocyte precursors develop in the neural crest and, as the embryo transitions into a human fetus, these melanocyte precursors migrate from the neural crest tissue to their permanent residence primarily in the skin. In the skin (and elsewhere in the body), the melanocytes retain some traces of their neural crest "disguise." The human immune system is tasked with the constant surveillance of cells within tissue and should identify cells that are out of place. The origin of the melanocyte in neural tissue allows it, when in its neoplastic form, to move through the body undetected by these sentinels of the immune system. This ability to migrate is the primary reason melanoma is such an aggressive and mortal cancer.

Melanocytes naturally reside primarily in the basement membrane of the epidermis. It is their role to generate small pigment packets, called melanosomes, which are placed in the surrounding epidermal cells. Much like the black paint used by athletes to draw the light from their eyes, the melanosome absorbs the energy of ultraviolet (UV) radiation before it hits the nucleus of the host cell. The ratio of melanocytes to basal cells varies significantly. Through a lifetime of exposure to UV radiation, a body generates more melanocytes to compensate for the increased exposure.

As the amount of UV exposure and the compensatory ratio of melanocytes to basal cells increases, so does the number of melanocytic lesions, melanoma precursors, and the risk of melanoma. Hence race/inherited skin types and the amount of UV exposure over a lifetime are the primary risk factors of melanoma. Those with more than 50 nevi or with atypical nevi are also at risk of melanoma. It is important to note the potential role of diet, UV blocking agents, and inherited gene mutations in that risk. There remains much to be learned about these risks and the role of nevi in the development of melanoma.

INTRODUCTION TO NEVI

Generally, nevi are clusters or growths of melanocytes. They are categorized by the location of the cluster of melanocytes in the dermis or epidermis, their presence at birth or developing after birth, and some clinical features. The majority of moles are acquired and sun exposure increases their frequency.

A quick and simplified review of the anatomy of the skin is helpful when considering the related terminology. The skin consists of the dermis (deeper layer, pink in **Fig. 1**) and epidermis (outer layer, purple in **Fig. 1**). The epidermis is nonvascular and is relatively thin, although its thickness varies by body site. The dermis makes up the majority of the skin's volume and is a complex network of vessels, nerves, follicles, and glands within a collagen matrix. These 2 layers are connected by an interlocking wavy layer

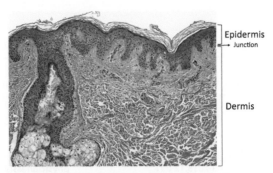

Epidermis
Junction

Dermis

Fig. 1. Histologic view of the skin showing the layers of interest.

(dermal papillae) at the "junction" of the epidermis and dermis labeled in **Fig. 1**. On the epidermal side of this junction, there is a layer of basal cells that gives rise to the epidermis. Melanocytes normally reside in a single layer interspersed throughout the basal cells.

Types of Nevi

- *Intradermal nevus*: these are usually raised flesh colored or pigmented lesions that arise from a cluster of melanocytes within the dermis (**Fig. 2**).
- *Junctional nevus*: these are usually flat and pigmented. They arise from the junction of the dermis and epidermis (**Fig. 3**).
- *Compound nevus*: mixes the features of an intradermal nevus and junctional nevus and arise from clusters of cells within both layers. They are usually pigmented and may be slightly raised with a surrounding flat pigmented area.
- *Blue nevus*: these are generally small black or dark blue lesions. The cluster of melanocytes that give rise to these lesions is deeper in the dermis giving it the appearance of being blue or black.
- *Congenital nevus*: small pigmented lesion that is present at birth or that develop in the first 2 years of life.
- *Giant congenital nevus*: these lesions are usually darkly pigmented and cover a large portion of the skin. They have a high propensity of developing melanoma but are very difficult to treat because of their size. They are also known as a bathing trunk nevus.
- *Spitz nevus*: this is a nevus of children or young adults that can be pink (classic Spitz) or pigmented. It has spindle-shaped cells and therefore is also referred to as a spindle cell nevus or epithelioid nevus

Many patients develop 1 or more "signature" patterns in the appearance of their nevi.[1] In essence, this means that they have multiple lesions with similar appearances. Some common patterns include:

- Brown or pink nevi
- Areas of hypopigmentation within the nevi
- Hypopigmented skin surrounding multiple nevi (halo pattern)
- Fried egg appearance where there is a darker round center (yolk) with a lighter periphery (egg white)

Although the appearance of these lesions can be concerning clinically, the presence of multiple lesion with similar patterns can be reassuring.

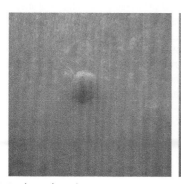 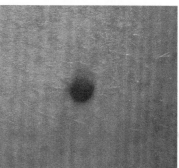

Fig. 2. Intradermal nevi.

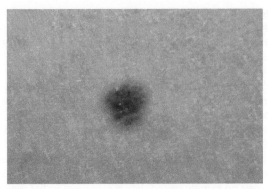

Fig. 3. Junctional nevus.

Treatment: When to Biopsy?

The bottom line when evaluating pigmented lesions is when and how to perform a biopsy. It is likely that this is where medicine truly becomes an art and a science. The art is knowing when to biopsy and how to biopsy adequately with minimal scarring or disfigurement. It is likely easier to balance an adequate and aesthetic aim than it is to know when a biopsy is necessary. That being said, there are newer more scientific methods available with varying degrees of support that help decide when a biopsy is warranted.

As discussed in the melanoma review, the ABCDEs (asymmetry, border irregularity, multiple or changing colors, large diameter, and evolution) of pigmented lesions are the traditional mantra. These criteria are certainly imperfect, because many benign pigmented lesions are considered outside the norm by their standards. Watching for evolution (change) and "the ugly duckling" may be a simple way to screen for melanomas. The downside of this method is the need to have multiple visits and the assistance of a knowledge of what the lesion looked like at baseline. Newer photography and computer-based models can be used as well.

Goodson and colleagues[2] recommend full body photography (mole mapping) as a viable way to screen for melanoma. Where time and resources allow, this method is certainly helpful. A sentinel review published by the same author gives a thorough review of nevi and their risk.[3] In this paper, it is noted that the risk of a nevus morphing into melanoma is 1 in 200,000 per year. The majority of melanomas were "de novo" arising from previously normal skin and not from preexisting nevi.[4]

As mentioned, the decision to biopsy or observe a lesion is complex. In some cases, patients with a history of skin cancer or melanoma insist on biopsies being performed. In other cases, lesions concerning for malignancy are found on patients who are reticent to have a biopsy done. A clinician must also consider social and historical factors. These might include, among others:

- Risk factors for melanoma
- Ability to follow-up and access to care
- Scars in cosmetically sensitive areas
- Age and health of the patient
- Cost

A simple approach in patients with extensive nevi or who are at high risk might be to identify the most clinically atypical lesions for biopsy at the first visit. These biopsies can serve as a baseline and spur a more aggressive approach if irregular or malignant or a more conservative approach if they are benign. Photography can be helpful when used by those trained in using baseline photographs as a clinical aid. Finally, a short interval between the first visit and follow-up visit (ie, 3–4 months) is useful to make sure nothing is changing rapidly. The following discussion details this process.

Treatment: Dysplastic Nevi

Biopsy results from pigmented lesions span an array from benign nevus to melanoma. In the middle of this spectrum are the "mild," "moderate," and "severely" dysplastic nevi. The decision to excise or not should take into consideration the involvement of the margins, severity of dysplasia, and clinical absence or presence of residual pigment. A recent retrospective review of excisions from mild and moderately dysplastic nevi showed little benefit in this additional surgery.[5] The recommendations are mixed in moderate to severely dysplastic lesions but more melanomas were found among the severely dysplastic nevi reexcisions.[6,7]

With the currently available data, it seems prudent to reexcise moderate and severely dysplastic lesions. However, each situation should be evaluated individually and consider more than just the pathologic diagnosis. In many situations, pathologists and dermatopathologists are helpful resources and willing to discuss the diagnosis and treatment.

Conclusions on Nevi

Although there is no clear consensus on screening intervals and methods, there is a vast amount of knowledge in the published literature. It seems that the importance of understanding each patients risk is paramount and must be considered when deciding on biopsy and treatment. Technological aids (photography, dermoscopy) can be helpful if properly used by clinicians with appropriate experience. Last, consultation with a specialist including the pathologist or dermatopathologist is useful.

MELANOMA

Melanoma is a malignancy of the melanocytes, or pigment-producing cells, of the body. It can be found on any skin or mucosal tissue, in the lymph nodes, and in the meninges. It is considered the most aggressive of all types of skin cancer. Melanoma can metastasize and be fatal if not treated aggressively. The National Cancer Institute predicted there would be roughly 75,000 newly diagnosed cases in 2015, more than doubling the number of new melanoma cases seen 40 years ago.[8,9] The rate of melanoma continues to increase steadily and the 2015 predicted melanoma-related deaths (just under 10,000) remains steady. Melanoma accounts for 1.7% of all cancer related deaths and three-quarters of all skin cancer deaths in the United States.[9,10] Malignant melanoma is found most often on the back and lower leg of women and on the back in men, although it can be found on any sun-exposed or non–sun-exposed part of the body. The recent diagnosis of former US president Jimmy Carter with melanoma in his liver and brain and no identifiable skin melanoma has brought "melanoma from an unknown primary" to the lime light. Although rare, having metastatic melanoma and no skin lesion accounts for about 3% of new melanoma diagnoses.[11]

Types of Melanoma

There are multiple types of melanoma based on growth pattern and location of origin[12]:

- Superficial spreading melanoma
- Lentigo maligna (typically occurs on skin-exposed sun where lentigines are likely to be found)
- Acral melanoma (occurs on palms, soles, and nail beds; most common type of melanoma in African Americans)
- Nodular melanoma
- Amelanotic melanoma (without pigment; often presents as pink papule or pink scaly plaque)
- Mucosal melanoma
- Neurotropic and desmoplastic melanoma (fibrous tumor with a tendency to grow down nerves)
- Ocular melanoma

Screening Guidelines

Current skin cancer screening recommendations differ by source. The US Preventive Services Task Force did not find evidence for or against regular screening by primary care clinicians.[13] The American Cancer Society has previously advocated for a full skin examination every 3 years in those aged 20 to 40 and every year for those over the age of 40.[8] Recently collected data argue that earlier detection through screening results in better survival.[14] These public health data do not, however, establish screening intervals or target populations. Patients with a history of melanoma should typically be followed very closely depending on stage. Screening guidelines for melanoma patients from the National Comprehensive Cancer Network recommend the following[15]:

- Stage 0: at least annually
- Stage I-IIA: every 6 to 12 months for 5 years then annually
- Stage IIB or higher: every 3 to 6 months for 2 years, then 3 to 12 for 3 years, then annually

Monthly self-skin examinations may be recommended between office visits to monitor for new lesions or changes in existing moles. The evidence for self-skin examinations is strongest in men and the elderly.[14] A truly complete full skin examination, including the scalp, feet, and genitals, is imperative in the early detection of melanoma.

Clinical Signs

Melanoma is typically asymptomatic and found on routine skin examination. If symptoms develop, they typically manifest as bleeding, itching, or pain.[8] The most commonly used mnemonic for evaluation of existing melanocytic lesions is the ABCDEs of melanoma, which has been an important message to primary care providers and patients promoting early melanoma detection (**Box 1**; ABCDs).

Evolution is often included as the "E" in the ABCDEs of melanoma mnemonic. Any change in texture, elevation, size, shape, color, or symptoms (bleeding, pain, itching) are important considerations when evaluating skin lesions as well. Although the ABCDEs of melanoma mnemonic can be helpful, it fails to include nodular melanoma, amelanotic melanoma, or those melanomas with a small diameter of 6 mm or less. Amelanotic melanoma and small diameter melanoma account for more than

---

Box 1
ABCDs of melanoma

A—Asymmetrical Shape

Melanoma lesions are often irregular, or not symmetric, in shape. If folded in half, a pigmented lesion should be a mirror image of itself.

B—Border

Typically, noncancerous moles have smooth, even borders. Melanoma lesions often have irregular borders that are difficult to define.

C—Color

The presence of more than 1 color (blue, black, brown, tan, etc) or the uneven distribution of color can sometimes be a warning sign of melanoma.

D—Diameter

Melanoma lesions are often greater than 6 mm in diameter (approximately the size of a pencil eraser).

Adapted from The Melanoma Research Foundation. Available at: www.melanoma.org. Accessed January 10, 2016.

---

one-half of all cases of reported melanoma, thus caution must be advised in the evaluation of skin lesions by providers without extensive dermatology experience.[16]

Another early melanoma detection tool developed in the 1980s is the Glasgow 7-point checklist. It consists of 7 features with that can be indicative of melanoma. Lesions exhibiting at least 3 of 7 are considered more at risk[16] (**Box 2**).

One other tool often considered in screening for melanoma is the "ugly duckling" sign. Most individuals with multiple nevi exhibit a common pattern or "signature nevus." Melanoma in these patients often presents as a nevus with features deviating from the typical nevi pattern.[17] Although none of these screening tools can be relied on solely for detection of melanoma, they are certainly good guidelines to consider when evaluating pigmented lesions.

Melanoma and Genetics

Although melanoma rates increase with UV exposure from the sun and indoor tanning devices, there is often a genetic component as well. One of the most significant risk factors for melanoma is a family history of the diagnosis. Familial cases of melanoma have been linked to 2 susceptibility genes, CDKN2A and CDK4.[18] Between 5% and

---

Box 2
Glasgow melanoma 7-point checklist

1. Sensory change (pain, itching, or other symptoms)
2. Diameter >7 mm
3. Irregular borders
4. Irregular pigmentation
5. Inflammation
6. History of lesion growth
7. Crusting, bleeding, oozing

10% of cutaneous melanoma is considered to be hereditary and related to mutations in these genes. CDKN2A mutations have been shown in families with 3 or more members diagnosed with melanoma, individuals with 3 or more primary melanomas, young age at diagnosis of melanoma, and the presence of both pancreatic cancer and melanoma in at least 1 family member.[19] Patients with any of these criteria in their family history should be counseled regarding the increased risk for melanoma, scheduled for regular skin cancer screenings, and educated on proper self-skin examinations for early detection of new or changing lesions.

Ultraviolet Exposure and Melanoma

UV light exposure greatly increases the risk of developing malignant melanoma, especially in those with fair skin, light eyes, blond or red hair, multiple nevi, or a family history of melanoma and dysplastic nevi. Any activity related to tan seeking, either via natural sunlight or tanning bed exposure, greatly increases the risk of melanoma. Patients with a history of first tanning bed exposure before age 30 have a 75% increased risk of developing melanoma in their lifetime.[20] In 2014, the US Food and Drug Administration reclassified sunlamp products to upgrade the carcinogenic risk level to moderate and added a black box warning contraindicating use in persons under the age of 18.[21] There has been important legislative work across the United States to ban or restrict tanning bed use in minors in an effort to combat this alarming trend. Although sun exposure before age 18 is an important risk factor for melanoma and nonmelanoma skin cancer, all exposure throughout a person's lifetime has a cumulative effect on increasing these risks. Proper daily sun protection and avoiding sun exposure during peak hours of UV radiation are key in reducing lifetime risk of melanoma in patients of all skin types.

Diagnosis

Diagnosis of cutaneous melanoma is obtained through skin biopsy. When taking a biopsy of a lesion suspicious for melanoma, it is important include the entire pigmented lesion to allow for appropriate determination of tumor thickness and subsequent staging and treatment.[22] Because Breslow depth, or tumor thickness, is the most important prognostic factor in predicting melanoma metastasis and survival, it is imperative that the biopsy go deep enough to avoid transecting the lesion at its base. Determination of diagnostic radiology screening, size of surgical margins, need for sentinel lymph node biopsy, and requirement for additional therapy beyond surgical excision all depend on the Breslow depth obtained from tumor thickness.[23] When possible, a full-thickness excisional biopsy should be performed when melanoma is suspected.

Staging

Tumor thickness of a primary melanoma is the most reliable prognostic factor in predicting the course of the malignancy.[24] Early diagnosis and timely surgery are imperative in melanoma management and favorable long term outcomes. The staging system for melanoma is based on the "TNM" (tumor, node, metastasis) system. Tumor thickness, ulceration, mitotic rate, lymph node involvement, and presence of metastasis are the important prognosticators. The American Joint Commission on Cancer's TNM staging method for melanoma is simplified[25] in **Table 1**.

Treatment Options

The ultimate goal for treatment of melanoma is surgical removal of the primary tumor with clear lateral and deep margins. Melanoma found before lymph node metastasis

Table 1
Clinical staging of Melanoma

Stage	T	N	M
0	Melanoma in situ	No lymph node involvement	No metastases present
IA	Primary lesion ≤1 mm depth without ulceration or mitoses	No lymph node involvement	No metastases present
IB	Primary lesion ≤2 mm without ulceration or ≤1 mm in depth, with ulceration, or ≥1 mitotic figure per mm²	No lymph node involvement	No metastases present
II	Primary lesion 1–2 mm with ulceration or ≤4 mm depth with or without ulceration	No lymph node involvement	No metastases present
III	Primary lesion of any size, regardless of ulceration	≥1 lymph node involved	No distant metastases present
IV	Primary lesion of any size, regardless of ulceration	Any number of lymph nodes involved	Metastases present

have a 5-year survival rate of about 80%, whereas those with lymphatic invasion have only a 50% 5-year survival rate.[26] Melanoma metastasis beyond the lymph nodes is often fatal within 9 months, with a 3-year survival rate of only 15%.[26] Current treatment guidelines for surgical margins in wide local excision of melanoma are based on Breslow depth at the time of diagnosis[15,27] (**Table 2**).

Malignant melanoma with metastases requires additional treatment beyond surgical excision. Sentinel lymph node biopsy is standard for all patients with melanoma greater than 1 mm deep and should be considered for tumors less than 1 mm in depth when there is an increased mitotic rate, ulceration, lymphovascular invasion, or extension of the tumor to the deep margin of the biopsy.[15] Sentinel lymph node biopsy involves injection of radioactive dye at the melanoma site before local tissue massage to enhance lymphatic drainage and localization of nodes involved in the area. Any nodes with radiotracer activity are removed and sent to pathology for evaluation.

Adjunctive therapy for advanced stage melanoma has been used with varying success in long-term survival rates. These treatments consist of chemotherapy, radiation therapy, and immunotherapy. Targeted immunotherapy is often used in cases where genetic mutations are thought to influence the behavior of melanoma. Immunotherapy in melanoma is aimed at manipulating the immune system of the patient or the tumor to combat these mutations. Immunotherapy is currently performed via use of interferons, interleukin-2, and a monoclonal antibody, ipilimumab. Immunotherapy offers an opportunity for prolonged disease-free states and, in the case of ipilimumab, increased survival for patients who are typically faced with 3-year survival rates of less than 15%.[26] Continued research is imperative to offer more treatment options

Table 2
Excision margins for melanoma

Breslow Depth	Excision Margin (cm)
Melanoma in situ	0.5–1
<2 mm	1
>2 mm	2

for the advanced stages of melanoma that are often fatal in an increasingly younger population.

Novel epigenetic therapies targeting the melanocyte signaling pathway are among the most promising treatment possibilities. Interrupting the melanocyte signaling pathway at the BRAF locus has shown improvement in survival.[28] Adding an interrupter at the MEK locus may block the tumors that circumvent the BRAF treatment.[29,30] Finally the PD1 molecule (programmed cell death) is being evaluated in many tumors and seems to have activity in treating melanoma.[31] It seems apparent that continued research along these epigenetic pathways will lead into the future of melanoma treatment.

SUMMARY

The spectrum of melanocytic lesions from nevi to melanoma is complex and requires attention to detail. In all cases, close and frequent observation by someone experienced in evaluating these lesions is best. There are numerous approaches and new technologies that can help diagnose, treat, and follow melanocytic lesions, but these must be used carefully because the experience of the operator clinician is the enabling or limiting factor.

REFERENCES

1. Suh KY, Bolognia JL. Signature nevi. J Am Acad Dermatol 2009;60(3):508–14.
2. Goodson AG, Florell SR, Hyde M, et al. Comparative analysis of total body and dermatoscopic photographic monitoring of nevi in similar patient populations at risk for cutaneous melanoma. Dermatol Surg 2010;36(7):1087–98.
3. Goodson AG, Grossman D. Strategies for early melanoma detection: approaches to the patient with nevi. J Am Acad Dermatol 2009;60(5):719–35 [quiz: 736–18].
4. Goodson AG, Florell SR, Boucher KM, et al. A decade of melanomas: identification of factors associated with delayed detection in an academic group practice. Dermatol Surg 2011;37(11):1620–30.
5. Strazzula L, Vedak P, Hoang MP, et al. The utility of re-excising mildly and moderately dysplastic nevi: a retrospective analysis. J Am Acad Dermatol 2014;71(6): 1071–6.
6. Reddy KK, Farber MJ, Bhawan J, et al. Atypical (dysplastic) nevi: outcomes of surgical excision and association with melanoma. JAMA Dermatol 2013;149(8): 928–34.
7. Abello-Poblete MV, Correa-Selm LM, Giambrone D, et al. Histologic outcomes of excised moderate and severe dysplastic nevi. Dermatol Surg 2014;40(1):40–5.
8. Pluta RM, Burke AE, Golub RM. JAMA patient page. Melanoma. JAMA 2011; 305(22):2368.
9. Seer Stat Factsheets. Melanoma of the skin. 2015. Available at: http://seer.cancer. gov/statfacts/html/melan.html. Accessed August 22, 2015.
10. Centers for Disease Control and Prevention (CDC). Deaths from melanoma – United States, 1973-1992. MMWR Morb Mortal Wkly Rep 1995;44(17):337, 343–347.
11. Katz KA, Jonasch E, Hodi FS, et al. Melanoma of unknown primary: experience at Massachusetts General Hospital and Dana-Farber Cancer Institute. Melanoma Res 2005;15(1):77–82.
12. DermNet NZ. Melanoma. 1997. Available at: www.dermnetnz.org/lesions/ melanoma.html. Accessed August 22, 2015.

13. US Preventive Services Task Force. Counseling to prevent skin cancer: recommendations and rationale of the U.S. Preventive services task force. MMWR Recomm Rep 2003;52(RR-15):13–7.
14. Curiel-Lewandrowski C, Chen SC, Swetter SM. Screening and prevention measures for melanoma: is there a survival advantage? Curr Oncol Rep 2012; 14(5):458–67.
15. National Comprehensive Cancer Network (NCCN). Melanoma guidelines. 2015;3(2015).
16. Tsao H, Olazagasti JM, Cordoro KM, et al. Early detection of melanoma: reviewing the ABCDEs. J Am Acad Dermatol 2015;72(4):717–23.
17. Grob JJ, Bonerandi JJ. The 'ugly duckling' sign: identification of the common characteristics of nevi in an individual as a basis for melanoma screening. Arch Dermatol 1998;134(1):103–4.
18. Hayward NK. Genetics of melanoma predisposition. Oncogene 2003;22(20): 3053–62.
19. Gabree M, Patel D, Rodgers L. Clinical applications of melanoma genetics. Curr Treat Options Oncol 2014;15(2):336–50.
20. Gandini S, Autier P, Boniol M. Reviews on sun exposure and artificial light and melanoma. Prog Biophys Mol Biol 2011;107(3):362–6.
21. U.S. Food and Drug Administration (FDA). Indoor tanning raises risk of melanoma: FDA strengthens warnings for sunlamp products. 2014. Consumer update. Available at: www.fda.gov/ForConsumers/ConsumerUpdates/ucm350790.htm. Accessed August 22, 2015.
22. Swanson NA, Lee KK, Gorman A, et al. Biopsy techniques. Diagnosis of melanoma. Dermatol Clin 2002;20(4):677–80.
23. Moore P, Hundley J, Levine EA, et al. Does shave biopsy accurately predict the final Breslow depth of primary cutaneous melanoma? Am Surg 2009;75(5): 369–73 [discussion: 374].
24. Kopf AW, Rigel D, Bart RS, et al. Factors related to thickness of melanoma. Multifactorial analysis off variables correlated with thickness of superficial spreading malignant melanoma in man. J Dermatol Surg Oncol 1981;7(8):645–50.
25. American Joint Committee on Cancer (AJCC). Melanoma of the skin staging. 7th edition. Chicago: AJCC; 2009.
26. Porter M, Stallings J. Melanoma: a brief overview including established immunotherapy treatment options. Journal of Dermatology for Physician Assistants 2015; 9(2):20–3.
27. Eedy DJ. Surgical treatment of melanoma. Br J Dermatol 2003;149(1):2–12.
28. Chapman PB, Hauschild A, Robert C, et al. Improved survival with vemurafenib in melanoma with BRAF V600E mutation. N Engl J Med 2011;364(26):2507–16.
29. Johnson AS, Crandall H, Dahlman K, et al. Preliminary results from a prospective trial of preoperative combined BRAF and MEK-targeted therapy in advanced BRAF mutation-positive melanoma. J Am Coll Surg 2015;220(4):581–93.e1.
30. Long GV, Stroyakovskiy D, Gogas H, et al. Combined BRAF and MEK inhibition versus BRAF inhibition alone in melanoma. N Engl J Med 2014;371(20):1877–88.
31. Robert C, Schachter J, Long GV, et al. Pembrolizumab versus Ipilimumab in advanced melanoma. N Engl J Med 2015;372(26):2521–32.

Nonmelanoma Skin Cancers Diagnosis and Management

Renata M. Block, MMS, PA-C, SDPA, ISDPA, AAPA, IAPA

KEYWORDS

- Nonmelanoma skin cancer • Squamous cell carcinoma • Basal cell carcinoma
- Actinic keratosis

KEY POINTS

- Nonmelanoma skin cancers are common cancers that are becoming an epidemic in the United States typically arising from precancerous cells that may be a result of extensive UV radiation exposure as well as other factors.
- An approach to treatment includes early diagnosis along with preventive measures and multiple therapies after a diagnosis is made to prevent disfiguration and recurrence.
- Guidelines outlining the specific care protocols for actinic keratosis, basal cell carcinomas, and squamous cell carcinomas are important for the management and clinical outcomes of patients.
- Health care providers play a key role in education, prevention, detection and treatment of nonmelanoma skin cancers.

INTRODUCTION

Diagnosis of actinic keratosis (AK) and nonmelanoma skin cancers can cost insurance companies billions of dollars every year. This largely preventable disease is actually growing in number instead of declining. With the popularity of indoor tanning being approved by the Food and Drug Administration (FDA) in 1978 and growing into a billion-dollar industry, the dermatologist has a challenge in convincing patients of the dangers that UV radiation, whether indoors or out, can cause. In addition to educating the patient that chronic cumulative exposure and sun burns are major risk factors, it is important to inform patients that there are other causes as well. The regular use of sunscreen, including reapplication, prevents the development of precancerous AK and results in regression of existing keratosis.[1] This may pose a challenge to the provider because in 2009 the average number of tanning salons exceeded the number of Starbucks and McDonalds in the United States.[2] However, as mentioned, other factors can play a key role in developing AK, basal cell carcinoma

Disclosure: None.
Pinski Dermatology & Cosmetic Surgery, S.C, 150 North Michigan Avenue, Suite 1200, Chicago, IL 60601, USA
E-mail address: rblock@dermpa.org

(BCC), and squamous cell carcinoma (SCC). These include but are not limited to family history and genetics (fair skin; blond/red hair; blue, green, gray eyes); also at risk are organ transplant recipients because of the therapy patients receive to prevent organ transplant rejections, and patients with low immune systems, whether from illness such as human immunodeficiency virus or AIDS or treatment modalities, like biologics and chemotherapies, for other diseases (**Box 1**). Because the precursor of most non-melanoma skin cancer is known as AK, for simplicity, AK is included in this discussion as a nonmelanoma skin cancer; however, it is known as a premalignancy.

Nonmelanoma skin cancers are most commonly derived from keratinocytes, an epidermal cell that synthesizes keratin and other proteins and sterols, with most cases of AK, BCC, and SCC evolving on the face, with one-half presenting on the nose.[3] Other common areas include the ears, scalp, neck, decollate, shoulders, arms, and legs; however, they can present in areas that are not exposed to sun. Providers look for all new or changing lesions, which are then deemed suspicious and evaluate if the lesion presents as an AK, BCC, and/or SCC; as all these types of growths can be seen in the same location and diagnosed from one lesional biopsy. Depending on the clinical suspicion of a lesion, to make a histologic diagnosis, a biopsy with a curette, punch, or dermablade is the diagnostic test of choice; these biopsies are simple, fast, and definitive.[3] Depending on the pathology-proven diagnosis, a treatment plan is derived. Most nonmelanoma skin cancers have a high cure rate with early diagnosis, and treatment.[4] Patient education is always provided at every office visit and information is provided for the patient to take home.

WHERE IT ALL BEGINS: THE EPIDERMIS

The skin has 3 distinct layers that are identified with the most superficial layer known as the epidermis. Keratinocytes make up 95% of the skin cells that are found in the epidermal layer and form distinct layers that are used for protection. The 4 layers include the following: stratum corneum (horny layer), stratum granulosum (granular layer), stratum spinulosum (spinous, spiny, or prickle cell layer), and stratum basale (basal layer) (**Fig. 1**). As they mature, keratinocytes differentiate into these 4 layers and accumulate keratin as they move outward, which takes approximately 22 days and is known as "epidermal renewal time."[5] This layer of the skin is superficial to the dermal layer. The subcutis layer is the third, deepest, layer of the skin (**Fig. 2**).

AK, BCC, and SCC all arise from keratinocytes. With the risk of 10% of AKs turning into SCCs, it is imperative to treat AKs to reduce the risk. They are recognized as pre-cancerous lesions and are common skin growths.[6] It is also now believed that some BCCs can arise from AKs as well. Approximately 65% of all SCCs and 36% of all BCCs arise in lesions that previously were diagnosed as AKs,[7] which makes the treatment of these precancerous lesions a priority with every patient visit. In 2009, the

---

Box 1
Risk factors for developing nonmelanoma skin cancers

1. UV radiation: Indoor and outdoor, cumulative exposure, or sunburns and/or long-term x-ray therapy.

2. Family history: Immediate blood relatives.

3. Genetic makeup: Fair skin, blond/red hair, blue/green/gray eyes.

4. Organ transplant recipients: Therapies to prevent organ rejection.

5. Low immune systems: Secondary to illness or treatment modalities of other diseases.

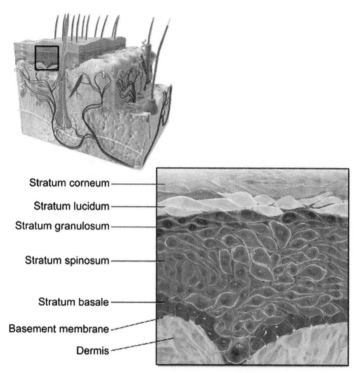

Fig. 1. The structure of the epidermis. (*From* Blausen.com staff. Blausen gallery 2014. Wikiversity Journal of Medicine. http://dx.doi.org/10.15347/wjm/2014.010.)

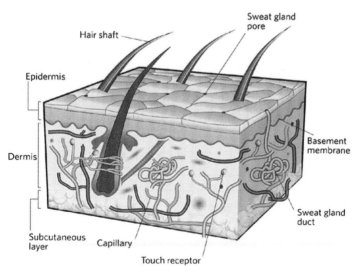

Fig. 2. Layers of the skin. (*From* MacNeil S. Review article progress and opportunities for tissue-engineered skin. Nature 2007;445(7130):875; with permission.)

1-year and 4-year risk of progression of AK into a malignant transformation in the Veterans Affairs Topical Tretinoin Chemoprevention Trial from baseline lesions was demonstrated. It is important to note that the rate of malignant transformation did not differ from the control group, and baseline AKs had significantly greater risk of progression to primary SCC invasive or in situ; $P = .2$[7,8] (**Table 1**).

AK is characterized by dysplasia and architectural disorder of the epidermis.[9] This premalignant cell of origin is the keratinocyte and under histology the epidermal layer is typically seen with hyperkeratosis and parakeratosis along with nuclear atypia of the keratinocyte, altered polarity, and can be found in the basal layer of the epidermis. Irregular acanthosis may be present (**Fig. 3**). It is usually not seen within hair follicles, sebaceous glands, or apocrine and eccrine ducts, which are located in the dermal layer. However, apocrine and eccrine glands can arise into the epidermis.[5] Even though AK, BCC, and SCC originate in the epidermis, histologically they can differ (**Table 2**). AK is now defined as the earliest clinical state in a continuum of malignancy that may progress to SCC in situ and/or invasive SCC, and also serves an important biological marker for field cancerization.[10–12]

Insurance and FDA-approved treatment in the office, therefore, is focused to the epidermis by ways of liquid nitrogen being the most common, along with photodynamic therapy (PDT) and surgical destruction of the lesion via curettage, shave, and excision. Even though cosmetic resurfacing procedures can play an important role in the treatment of AKs (medium, deep chemical peels, dermabrasion, and ablative laser), these are not billable to insurance because of their cosmetic nature. Therefore, the treatment in the office may take a multifactorial approach, but the patient may be responsible for some of the cost.

Topical medications, known as "field therapy," approved by the FDA for the treatment of AK include the following[13–15]: topical 5-fluorouracil (5-FU), topical diclofenac gel, imiquimod cream, and ingenol mebutate gel. These are known to treat both clinical and subclinical AKs. The following sections include, in order of FDA approval, the generic name (trade), mechanism of action (MOA), and side effects (SEs) for each of the topical medications (please see the package insert for full MOA and potential SEs listed for each drug).

Topical 5-Fluorouracil

FDA approval 1970s (Efudex, Fluoroplex, Carac cream 5%, 0.5%).

Mechanism of action

A topical chemotherapy that destroys AK by converting into specific nucleotides resulting into an antitumor effect by inhibiting thymidylate synthase, the rate-limiting

Table 1
Malignant transformation of AK in the Veterans Affairs Topical Tretinoin Chemoprevention Trial: risk of progression

Malignant Transformation	Risk of Progression at 1 y (95% CI), %	Risk of Progression at 4 y (95% CI), %
AK to Primary SCC	0.60 (0.44–0.82)	2.57 (2.12–3.12)
AK to Primary Invasive SCC	0.39 (0.26–0.57)	1.97 (1.58–2.47)
AK to Primary BCC	0.48 (0.34–0.68)	1.56 (1.21–2.02)
AK to any KC (SCC or BCC)	1.08 (0.85–1.36)	4.10 (3.53–4.77)

Abbreviations: AK, actinic keratosis; BCC, basal cell carcinoma; CI, confidence interval; KC, keratinocyte carcinoma; SCC, squamous cell carcinoma.
  Data from Geng A, Weinstock MA, Hall R, et al. Veterans Affairs Topical Tretinoin Chemoprevention Trial. Br J Dermatol 2009;161(4):918–24

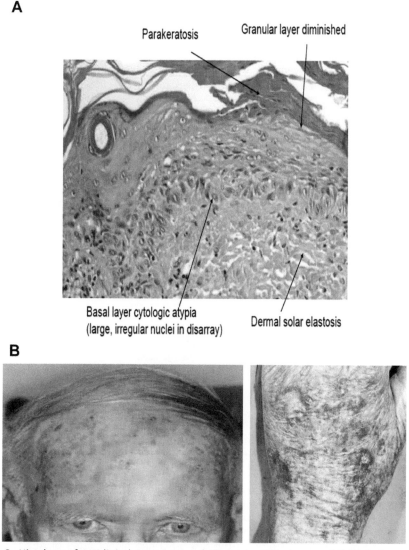

A

Parakeratosis

Granular layer diminished

Basal layer cytologic atypia
(large, irregular nuclei in disarray)

Dermal solar elastosis

B

Fig. 3. Histology of AK/clinical appearance of AKs and actinic damage. (*A*) Clinical appearance of AK (hematoxylin-eosin, original magnification ×400). (*B*) Actinic damage with multiple AKs to the forehead and left hand. (*From* Rapini RP. Practical dermatopathology. Philadelphia: Elsevier Mosby; 2005; with permission.)

enzyme in the pyrimidine nucleotide synthesis.[16] As a result, this thymine deficiency interferes with DNA synthesis and formation of RNA, which are essential for cell division and growth. This deficiency stops the growth of rapidly proliferating or cancerous cells and eventually results in death of that cell.

Side effects Pregnancy Category X and general adverse events (AEs) occur locally and are considered to be drug-related and occur with frequency: erythema, dryness, pruritus, burning, crusting, erosion, ulceration, pain, edema.[17]

Table 2
Difference between AK, BCC, SCC (cSCC)

Pre- and Nonmelanoma Types of Skin Cancer	Originates in Epidermis	Histology	Affected Areas
1. Actinic keratosis (AK)[a]	Premalignant cell of origin: Keratinocyte.	Hyperkeratosis/parakeratosis of epidermis, nuclear atypia, abnormal keratinocytes of the basal layer, altered polarity, irregular acanthosis may be present.	Epidermis only and not affected in hair follicles, sebaceous glands, apocrine and eccrine ducts.
2. Basal cell carcinoma (BCC)	Cell of origin: Keratinocyte. Arise from pluripotential cells in basal layer of epidermis or follicular structures.	Solid cellular strands, collection of cells with dark-staining large nuclei and scant cytoplasm.	Found mainly in hair-bearing areas and rarely metastasize.
3. Cutaneous squamous cell carcinoma (cSCC)	Cell of origin: Keratinocyte. Apoptotic resistance through functional loss of TP53, a tumor suppressor gene.	Hyperkeratosis/parakeratosis, nuclear atypia, frequent mitosis, cellular pleomorphism, disorganized progression of cells from the basal to apical layers of the epidermis. Divided into 2 categories: cSCC in situ and invasive cSCC.	Small percentage can metastasize to lymph nodes, soft tissue, or bone.

[a] Premalignancy: Because the precursor of most nonmelanoma skin cancer is known as the AK.
   Data from Medscape.

Efficacy Monotherapy, at 4 weeks after treatment, complete clearance rates of 0.5% and 5% 5-FU ranged from 16.7% to 57.8% and 43% to 100%, respectively. In the only split-face study comparing both formulations, both treatments produced equivalent rates (43%) of complete clearance, but 5% 5-FU had higher rates of AEs.[18] One week usage of fluorouracil cream (0.5%) before cryosurgery has been shown to produce complete lesion clearance in more patients compared with cryosurgery alone (32.4% and 15%, respectively).[19]

Topical diclofenac gel
FDA approval 2000s (Solaraze gel 3%).

Mechanism of action A nonsteroidal anti-inflammatory drug that destroys AK, and is known to inhibit cyclooxygenase (specifically cyclooxygenase-2), which decreases prostaglandin production and reverses suppression of apoptosis and alters angiogenesis.

Side effects Pregnancy Category B. It produces little to no inflammation and thus is very well tolerated.[7] Application site reactions were the most frequent AEs that included contact dermatitis, rash, dry skin, and exfoliation.[20]

Efficacy Diclofenac therapy after cryosurgery also has been shown to produce complete lesion clearance in a large number of patients compared with cryosurgery alone (64% and 32%, respectively).[21]

Imiquimod cream
FDA approval 2004, 2010 (Aldara cream 5%, Zyclara cream 2.5%, 3.75%).

Mechanism of action Induces the body's own immune system to destroy AK. Also known as an immune response modifier that upregulates a variety of cytokines, which, in turn, invoke a nonspecific immune response (interferons, natural killer cells) and a specific immune response (T cells) that stimulates apoptosis.[7]

Side effects Pregnancy Category C. Flu symptoms, mild skin irritation (itching, dryness, scabbing), headache, dizziness, cold sores, nausea, diarrhea.[22]

Efficacy Lower formulations of 2.5% and 3.75% were found to be more efficacious than a 5% formulation, and clearance rates of 25% and 34% were found, respectively. However, approximately 44% of patients found complete clearance with the 5% cream.[22]

Ingenol mebutate gel
FDA approval 2012 (Picato gel 0.015%, 0.05%).

Mechanism of action Precise MOA has not been defined but described as a dual MOA, which includes a rapid necrosis by mitochondrial swelling and membrane disruption and specific neutrophil-mediated, antibody-dependent cellular cytotoxicity by antibodies produced from B cells that bind to antigens on dysplastic epidermal cells.[23]

Side effects Most common adverse reaction (AR) (>2%) resolved without sequelae were generally mild to moderate in intensity are local skin reactions, application site erythema, pain, pruritus, irritation, erosion/ulceration infection, periorbital edema, nasopharyngitis, and headache.

Efficacy Complete and partial clearance rates are 37% and 60%, respectively.
For the best results of management of AKs, it is best to use any of these prescribed topical therapies as "field therapy" in conjunction with an "ablative therapy," such as liquid nitrogen, PDT, and/or skin resurfacing (dermabrasion, chemical peeling, or laser resurfacing), which are done in the office setting. However, these augmented treatments may have to be repeated over time. Although both can result in some "down time" for each patient, using these therapeutic options synergistically can induce a more substantial clearance rate that is far more effective and economical than stand-alone treatments. This comprehensive management of AK should be based on the judgment of the clinician for the patient on a case-by-case basis.

BASAL CELL CARCINOMA

BCC is the most superficial and common form of nonmelanoma skin cancer and is usually caused by a cumulative and intense, occasional UV exposure from natural sunlight and tanning beds, specifically UVB (290–320 nm). It is also known to be caused by previous radiation treatments and because of genetic makeup and is found in those with low immunity and in organ transplant recipients. However, 90% of nonmelanoma skin cancers are attributed to exposure to UV radiation (indoor and/or outdoor), with BCC being most of this percentage, roughly 80%.[10] BCCs frequently develop on the face, neck, shoulders, back, scalp, and ears; however, it can develop in places that have not been exposed to much UV radiation and the tendency to develop a BCC also may be

Box 2
Basal cell carcinoma (BCC) histopathologic subtypes, clinical appearances, and DDX

Nodular BCC:

Histologic Presentation (**Fig. 4**A): Nodular BCCs account for half of all BCCs and are characterized by nodules of large basophilic cells and stromal retraction. The term micronodular is used to describe tumors with multiple microscopic nodules smaller than 15 μm.

Clinical Presentation (**Fig. 4**B): Most common clinical subtype of BCC. Commonly found on the sun-exposed areas of head and neck. Appears as a translucent papule or nodule. Usually telangiectasias and rolled border.

DDX: Traumatized dermal nevus, amelanotic melanoma, squamous cell carcinoma (SCC), fibrous papule of face, molluscum contagiosum, sebaceous hyperplasia.

Pigmented BCC:

Histologic Presentation (**Fig. 5**A): Pigmented BCC shows histologic features similar to those of nodular BCC but with the addition of melanin. Approximately 75% of BCCs contain melanocytes but only 25% contain large amounts of melanin. The melanocytes are interspersed between tumor cells and contain numerous melanin granules in their cytoplasm and dendrites. Although the tumor cells contain little melanin, numerous melanophages populate the stroma surrounding the tumor.

Clinical Presentation (**Fig. 5**B): Subtype of nodular BCC. Exhibits increased melanization. Appears as a hyperpigmented, translucent papule, which may also be eroded.

DDX: Nodular melanoma, melanocytic nevi, molluscum contagiosum, SK.

Superficial BCC:

Histologic Presentation (**Fig. 6**A): Superficial BCC is characterized microscopically by buds of malignant cells extending into the dermis from the basal layer of the epidermis. The peripheral cell layer shows palisading. There may be epidermal atrophy, and dermal invasion is usually minimal. This histologic subtype is encountered most often on the trunk and extremities but may also appear on the face and neck. There may be a chronic inflammatory infiltrate in the upper dermis.

Clinical Presentation (**Fig. 6**B): Occurs mostly on the trunk and appears as an erythematous patch (often well demarcated).

DDX: Eczema, psoriasis, actinic keratosis (AK), Bowen disease, SCC.

Morpheaform BCC:

Histologic Presentation (**Fig. 7**A): Also known as infiltrative BCC, consists of strands of tumor cells embedded within a dense fibrous stroma. Tumor cells are closely packed and, in some cases, only 1 cell thick.

Clinical Presentation (**Fig. 7**B): Aggressive growth variant of BCC with distinct clinical and histologic appearance. Ivory-white appearance, may resemble a scar or small lesion of morphea.

DDX: Localized scleroderma, scar tissue.

Fibroepithelioma of pinkus (FEP):

Histologic Presentation (**Fig. 8**A): In FEP, long strands of interwoven basiloma cells are embedded in fibrous stroma. Histologically, FEP shows features of reticulated seborrheic keratosis and superficial BCC.

Clinical Presentation (**Fig. 8**B): Pink papule, usually on the lower back.

DDX: Acrochordon, fibroma.

Metatypical:

Histologic Presentation (**Fig. 9**A): Intermediate typology between BCC and SCC. Possesses histologic features of both BCC and SCC. It has a higher rate of metastasis. Also known as basosquamous. Shows cytoplasmic keratinization and/or intercellular bridges in the squamous areas.

Clinical Presentation (**Fig. 9**B): Difficult to distinguish and needs a histologic diagnosis.

DDX: AK, SCC, SK

Abbreviations: DDX, diffential diagnosis; SK, seborrheic keratosis.
  Data from Wolff K, Goldsmith LA, Katz SI, et al, editors. Fitzpatrick's dermatology in general medicine. 7th edition. New York: McGraw-Hill; 2008. p. 1038–9.

inherited. BCCs tend to grow slowly and after years of growth by attaining a size of only 1 to 2 cm or more in diameter. This type of skin cancer is rarely fatal and can have an excellent prognosis, but can be highly disfiguring if allowed to grow.[24,25]

As discussed, it arises from the most superficial layer of the skin known as the epidermis. The cell of origin is the keratinocyte, specifically known as pluripotential cells, of the stratum basale (see **Fig. 1**), which is the basal layer of the epidermis. The pluripotential cells can also be found in follicular structures, which is why BCCs are found mainly in hair-bearing areas. Specifically, the pluripotent cell is a stem cell that can give rise to all tissue types (keratinocytes making up the epidermis), but not to an entire organism. With embryonic development, they continue to divide to further specialize into cell types.[26] This type of cancer is rarely known to metastasize, but fewer than 1% can grow deep into tissue and bone.[27] A BCC is best diagnosed based on various biopsy techniques, including a curette, punch, double-edged blade, or dermablade. The histology of BCCs may vary somewhat with subtype, but they are made up of solid cellular strands and a collection of cells with dark-staining large nuclei, which may not appear atypical, and scant cytoplasm[28] (see **Table 2**). Clinically, they can appear as a shiny and/or pink papule with telangiectasia, a growth resembling a scar that is white, yellow, or appears shiny; a friable, nonhealing lesion; or even a red patch of skin. An intradermal nevus without pigment on the face of older fair skinned individuals may resemble a BCC and a biopsy should be performed if this is a newly acquired growth. These are further divided into histopathological subtypes and clinical appearances (**Box 2**).[28,29]

Its histologic subtypes are divided into 2 categories: undifferentiated and differentiated. These are beyond the scope of this article, but should be recognized.

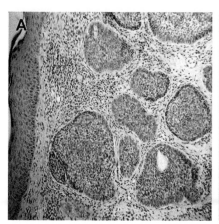
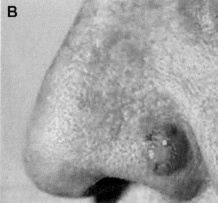

Fig. 4. (*A, B*) Nodular BCC. Hematoxylin-eosin, original magnification ×400. (*From* Practical dermatopathology 2005 & dermatology. 2nd edition. New York (US): Elsevier; 2008.)

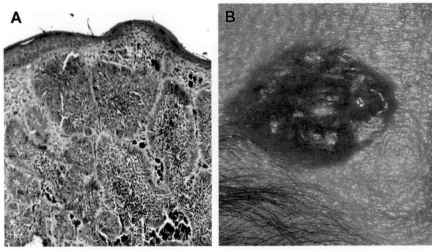

Fig. 5. (*A, B*) Pigmented BCC. (*From* Rapini RP. Practical dermatopathology. Philadelphia: Elsevier Mosby; 2005; with permission.)

Undifferentiated BCCs: Little or no differentiation and is referred to as a solid BCC. This includes superficial BCC, pigmented BCC, sclerosing BCC, and infiltrative BCC.

Differentiated BCCs: Most commonly diagnosed and often have a slight differentiation toward the following: hair (keratotic BCC), sebaceous glands (BCC with sebaceous differentiation), tubular glands (adenoid BCC), and noduloulcerative (nodular).[22]

Discussion of basal cell nevus syndrome is also beyond the scope of this article but it should be noted that it is known as nevoid BCC and Gorlin syndrome. This is a rare autosomal dominant disorder.

There are a variety of treatment modalities for BCC that a clinician can choose from, but the management should be on an individual case basis, such as patient factors and cost, as well as the size of the tumor, anatomic location, and histology. The treatment management can be surgical and nonsurgical (**Box 3**).[10,22,27,28]

It is important to note that (unlike Mohs surgery and excisional surgery), electrodessication and curettage (ED&C), radiation, cryosurgery, and topical medications all have one significant drawback in common because no tissue is examined under the microscope (with the exception of ED&C), so there is no way to determine how

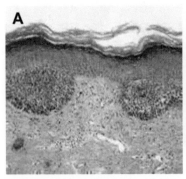

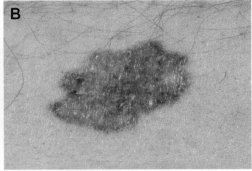

Fig. 6. (*A, B*) Superficial BCC. (*From* Practical dermatopathology 2005 & dermatology. 2nd edition. Elsevier; 2008.)

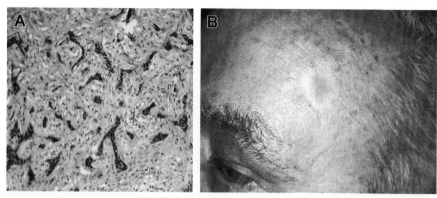

Fig. 7. (*A, B*) Morpheaform BCC. (*From* Rapini RP. Practical dermatopathology. Philadelphia: Elsevier Mosby; 2005; with permission.)

completely the tumor was removed.[24] The recurrence rates and risks of treatment must be accounted for when determining the proper management of BCC. Anatomic sites with a high risk of local recurrence in areas of important tissue conservation include the following: face, including the central one-third of the face, nose, nasolabial folds, and periorbital, perioral, and periauricular regions; hands, feet; and genitalia.[4] The prognosis is a 100% survival rate for cases that have not metastasized.

SQUAMOUS CELL CARCINOMA

SCC is the second most common form of nonmelanocytic skin cancer and accounts for approximately 16% of the 90% of nonmelanoma skin cancers that are attributed to UV radiation exposure. It is caused by a cumulative UV exposure over the course of a lifetime, including year-round exposure and intense exposure in the summer months. This includes radiation exposure to UVA (320–400 nm) and UVB (290–320 nm). The most common areas affected are those that are frequently exposed to the sun. This includes the rim of the ear, lower lip, face, scalp, neck, arms (including hands), and

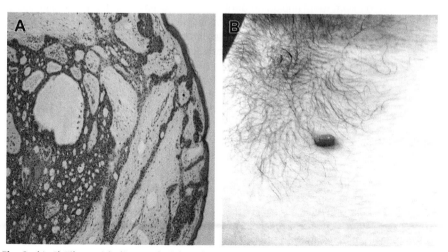

Fig. 8. (*A, B*) Fibroepithelioma of pinkus. (*From* Rapini RP. Practical dermatopathology. Philadelphia: Elsevier Mosby; 2005; with permission.)

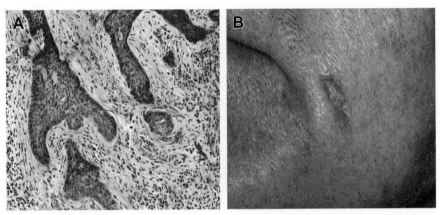

Fig. 9. (*A, B*) Metatypical. (*From* Rapini RP. Practical dermatopathology. Philadelphia: Elsevier Mosby; 2005; with permission.)

legs. However, SCC can occur in all areas of the body, including mucous membranes and the genitalia area. It is usually seen in individuals with fair skin; light hair; and blue, green, or gray eyes, as these patients are at the highest risk, but anyone with a history of substantial sun exposure is at increased risk of developing an SCC. It also has been found in people who have had a history of prolonged exposure to x-rays or certain chemicals. It is well documented that anyone with a previous history of BCC is at increased of developing an SCC. It should be noted that a highly UV-sensitive condition known as xeroderma pigmentosum increases a person's risk of developing an SCC; however, this condition is beyond the scope of this article.

It is best to detect this type of skin cancer at an early stage and have it removed promptly. SCCs are known to penetrate underlying tissue and a small percentage may metastasize to local lymph nodes, distant tissues, and organs, which can be fatal. The lesions are not as distinctive as a BCC and may be easily misdiagnosed clinically. SCC located in mucosal surfaces such as the lip, oral cavity, tongue, and genitalia have much higher rates of metastasis. Mucosal surface SCC may develop from chronic irritation from teeth (including dentures), a long-time habit of a biting injury inside the buccal mucosa or lip, and even habitual alcohol consumption or tobacco use (smoking or chewing). SCC may appear as small red, scaly thin plaques or red, keratotic (wartlike), conical hard nodules (cutaneous horns) that occasionally ulcerate (**Fig. 10**). They have a tendency to occur in skin that has been inflamed or injured, especially skin that has been scarred by burns.

SCCs arise from the main structural cells of the epidermis known as the keratinocytes. The epidermis is made up of protein cells called keratinocytes, also referred to as squamous cells. As in most cancers, the development of SCC from normal keratinocytes begins with mutations in the cellular DNA.[28] SCC results in keratinocytes not dividing in an orderly manner, which can spread deeper into the next layer of skin, the dermis, and become invasive to the surrounding tissue. Along the pathway to SCC, keratinocytes become resistant to apoptosis (programmed cell death) and immune attack.[28] The p53 tumor suppressor plays a large role in the protection against skin cancer cells by removing any cells that have acquired a mutation. This is specifically important because the p53 regulation, which delays cell cycle progression until DNA damage, can be repaired, are derived within the keratinocyte cell (see **Table 2**). Although, like BCC, they are slow growing, some can be very aggressive and spread to other parts of the body, including fat tissues, lymph nodes, and internal organs, and cause death.

Box 3
BCC surgical and nonsurgical treatment modalities

Surgical

Surgery (excisional surgery, Mohs, electrodesiccation and curettage [ED&C], cryosurgery): This is the best management and recommended treatment modality.

Excisional Surgery: Standard excision offers the removed specimen to be histologically evaluated. Excision should include extension into subcutaneous fat to ensure adequate tumor removal. *Cure rate*: More than 95%.

Mohs Micrographic Surgery: Surgical technique that is microscopically controlled for all types and sizes of BCC. Treatment of choice for poorly defined tumors or tumors with high recurrence rate. *Cure rate*: Highest cure rate at 99%.

ED&C: Most beneficial for nodular BCC smaller than 6 mm. *Cure rate*: 93% to 95% and may have to be repeated a few times.

Cryosurgery: Not indicated for tumors deeper than 3 mm. Best for elderly patients with bleeding disorders or intolerance to anesthesia. *Cure rate*: 85% to 90%, but not commonly used because it lacks confirmation of complete tumor removal.

Nonsurgical

Observation/No treatment: Usually in the elderly patient; however, close observation in these patients is warranted.

Radiation Therapy (RT): Best used when surgery is contraindicated, but can be used after surgery as an adjunct for aggressive tumors or difficulty with clearance of margins with surgery. *Cure rate*: Approximately 90%, but control rate of 93% has been reported.

Photodynamic Therapy (PDT) (as an adjunct): PDT is a treatment that uses aminolevulinic acid and exposure to wavelengths of light to produce a form of oxygen that kills nearby cells. This should be considered for elderly patients or tumor recurrence with tissue atrophy and scar formation or tumors with poorly defined borders based on clinical examination. Effective method of treating recurrent BCCs that are smaller than 1 cm. *Cure rate*: 88% clearance rate after 1 to 3 treatments for BCC larger than 2 cm.

Pharmacologic Therapy
5-FU: 5% Fluorouracil is a topical cytostatic agent and may be used to treat small, superficial BCCs in low-risk area. *Cure rate*: Generally more than 80% and 5-year recurrence rate of 21%.
Imiquimod: Is a topical cytostatic agent used to treat nonfacial superficial BCC. *Cure rate*: 75%.
Vismodegib (Erivedge): Oral agent, hedgehog pathway inhibitor, to treat advanced forms of BCC. Alterations in hedgehog signaling are implicated in the pathogenesis of BCC. *Cure rate*: Phase 1 study showed a 58% response rate and can be used before surgery to shrink large tumors. *Side effects*: Muscle spasms, alopecia, dysgeusia (taste disturbance), weight loss, and fatigue.[31]

Data from Wolff K, Goldsmith LA, Katz SI, et al, editors. Fitzpatrick's dermatology in general medicine. 7th edition. New York: McGraw-Hill; 2008. p. 1038–9.

SCC in situ, also known as Bowen disease, is the earliest form of SCC and can appear anywhere on the skin, including the mucosal surfaces (leukoplakia), and the lips, particularly the lower lip (actinic cheilitis). The cells are "in situ," meaning the cancer is in the epidermis and has not spread to the dermis (noninvasive). The appearance is usually an asymptomatic erythematous scaly thin plaque or white patch on mucosal surfaces, including the lip (**Fig. 11**). Perhaps the most common form of Bowen disease known is caused by the human papilloma virus, which is sexually transmitted and mostly found in the genital region, but can also be found in the mucous membranes of the mouth and nose as well as the skin. Histologically, characteristics include

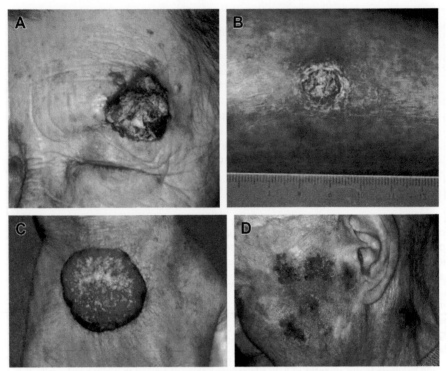

Fig. 10. Clinical spectrum of cutaneous squamous cell carcinoma (SCC). (*A*) A large keratotic nodule of the supraorbital region in an elderly woman; note the coarse wrinkling and solar elastosis of the face. (*B*) Eroded and keratotic nodule that developed rapidly at the site of trauma on the shin. (*C*) Large, fungating nodule on the dorsum of the hand. (*D*) Multiple eroded superficial SCCs in association with hypertrophic AKs on the cheek and neck of an elderly man. (*From* Soyer HP, Rigel DS, Wurm EMT. Actinic keratosis, basal cell carcinoma and squamous cell carcinoma. In: Bolognia JL, Jorizzo JL, Schaffer JV, eds. Dermatology. 3rd edition. Philadelphia: Elsevier, 2012; with permission.)

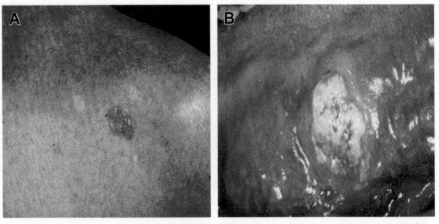

Fig. 11. (*A, B*) Bowen disease and leukoplakia. (*From* Rapini RP. Practical dermatopathology. Philadelphia: Elsevier Mosby; 2005; with permission.)

nuclear atypia, frequent mitoses, cellular pleomorphism, parakeratosis, and hyperkeratosis, as well as a disorganized progression of cells from the basal to apical layers of the epidermis[30] (**Fig. 12**). Treatment is necessary to avoid invasive growth. Treatment includes surgical excision, cryotherapy, PDT, and 5-FU cream.

Invasive SCC is a staged nonmelanoma skin cancer classified according to the American Joint Committee on Cancer/International Union against Cancer tumor-node-metastasis (TNM) staging system[31] (**Table 3**). There is an additional N1S3 staging system for metastatic SCC of the head and neck, but is beyond the scope of this article.[31] An SCC is best diagnosed based on a biopsy that should include a full-thickness representation via excision or punch of the skin so depth can be evaluated. Further evaluation by computed tomography scanning may be needed to rule out any bone, lymph node, or soft tissue invasion, and/or MRI, which is preferred for evaluation of perineural invasion and orbital or intracranial extension.[30] Clinically, these may appear as an AK, BCC, atopic or allergic contact dermatitis, verruca vulgaris, seborrheic keratosis, chemical burns, pyoderma gangrenosum, melanocytic nevus, trauma, or herpes simplex virus or varicella-zoster virus. Conventional cutaneous SCC (cSCC) can be divided into 3 histologic grades, based on the degree of nuclear atypia and keratinization found; however, due to histologic similarities of other diseases, special staining may be needed to establish a diagnosis (**Box 4**).

Treatment of SCC includes nonexcisional/nonsurgical management, such as 5-FU, imiquimod, PDT (in situ tumors and special circumstances, such as location, patient's age, intolerance to anesthetics). It also can be treated by ED&C, radiation therapy, surgical excision, and Mohs micrographic surgery. High-risk SCC should be recognized, as treatment is based on the characteristics of lesions (**Box 5**).

The choice of treatment is determined by several factors, including tumor type, size, location, and depth of penetration, as well as the patient's age and general health[24] (see **Box 4**; **Box 6**).

Treatment on SCC diagnosis is dependent of histologic grade, TNM staging, and category of risk. Nonetheless, it may take a multifactorial approach and should be based on each individual on a case-by-case basis.

THE ROLE OF SUNSCREEN

Because most AKs and nonmelanoma skin cancers can result from cumulative exposure to UV radiation, it is important to know the role of sunscreens as well as other

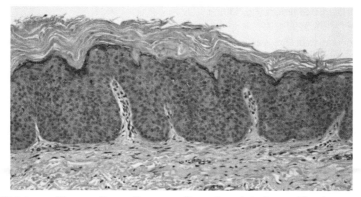

Fig. 12. Histology of Bowen disease (hematoxylin-eosin, original magnification ×100). (*From* Rapini RP. Practical dermatopathology. Philadelphia: Elsevier Mosby; 2005; with permission.)

Table 3
TNM staging for nonmelanoma skin cancer

T = Primary tumor	
T0	No evidence of primary tumor
Tis	Carcinoma in situ
T1	≤2 cm
T2	>2 cm
T3	Invasion of deep structures
T4	Direct or perineural invasion of skull base or axial skeleton
High-risk tumor features	
Depth/invasion	• 4-mm thickness • Clark level IV • Perineural invasion • Lymphovascular invasion
Anatomic location	• Primary site ear • Primary site nonglabrous lip
Differentiation	Poorly differentiated or undifferentiated
N = Regional lymph nodes	
N0	No regional lymph node metastasis
N1	Metastasis in a single lymph node, ≤3 cm
N2	Metastasis in a single lymph node, 3–6 cm or metastasis in multiple lymph nodes, ≤6 cm
N2	Metastasis in a lymph node >6 cm
M = Distant metastasis	
M0	No distant metastasis
M1	Distant metastasis

From UICC International Union against Cancer. Skin tumors. In: Sobin L, Gospodarowicz M, Wittekind C, editors. TNM classification of malignant tumors. West Sussex (United Kingdom): Wiley-Blackwell; 2010. p. 876; with permission.

Box 4
Cutaneous SCC (cSCC) histologic grades and variants

SCC histologic grades:

Well Differentiated: Characterized by more normal-appearing nuclei with abundant cytoplasm and extracellular keratin pearls (**Fig. 13**A).
   Histologic DDX: Verruca vulgaris, inverted follicular keratosis, seborrheic keratosis.

Moderately Differentiated: Exhibits features intermediate between well-differentiated and poorly differentiated lesions (**Fig. 13**B).
   Histologic DDX: Angiosarcoma, sebaceous carcinoma.

Poorly Differentiated: Shows a high degree of nuclear atypia with frequent mitoses, a greater nuclear-cytoplasmic ratio, and less keratinization; it may be difficult to distinguish from mesenchymal tumors, melanoma, or lymphoma (**Fig. 13**C).
   Histologic DDX: Atypical fibroxanthoma, fibrosarcoma, Merkel cell carcinoma, malignant melanoma (MM).

SCC histologic variants:

Aggressive Clinical SCC: Variants include acantholytic (adenoid) SCC, which is characterized by a pseudoglandular appearance, and spindle cell SCC, which has atypical, spindle-shaped cells (**Fig. 14**).

Keratoacanthoma (KA): This dome-shaped, large, smooth or verrucous nodule is not histologically an SCC, but is viewed as a clinical subtype of SCC. It is known to spontaneously resolve, however, and should be treated as an SCC (**Fig. 15**).

Data from Wolff K, Goldsmith LA, Katz SI, et al, editors. Fitzpatrick's dermatology in general medicine. 7th edition. New York: McGraw-Hill; 2008. p. 1038–9.

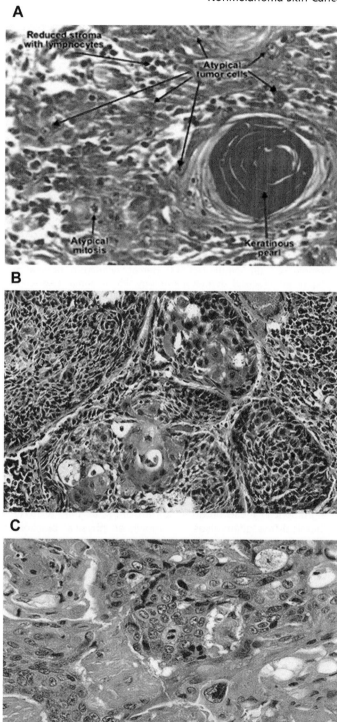

Fig. 13. (A) Histology of well-differentiated SCC. (B) Histology of moderately differentiated SCC. (C) Histology of poorly differentiated SCC. Hematoxylin-eosin, original magnification ×400. (*From* Rapini RP. Practical dermatopathology. Philadelphia: Elsevier Mosby; 2005; with permission.)

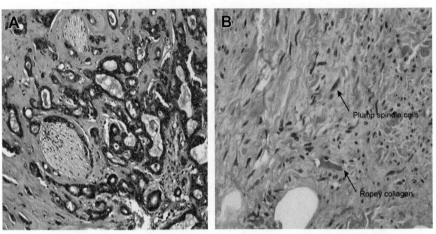

Fig. 14. (A) Adenoid SCC. (B) Spindle cell SCC. Hematoxylin-eosin, original magnification ×400. (*From* Rapini RP. Practical dermatopathology. Philadelphia: Elsevier Mosby; 2005; with permission.)

modalities used to prevent AKs, BCCs, and SCCs. Sunscreens with a sun protection factor (SPF) commenced in 1962 and not until 1978 were given an SPF rating of 15 that was regulated by the FDA. Its main purpose was to prevent sunburns which are mainly caused by UVB rays. It is an indication of how long it will take to develop a sunburn as compared with unprotected skin. For example, if it takes an individual 10 minutes to burn, an SPF 30 will allow that individual to be out for 300 minutes before burning (30 SPF × 10 minutes = 300 minutes). However, UVA is hugely responsible for the damage of the DNA within the skin causing premature aging, wrinkles, and skin cancers. This is not yet rated by the FDA but is recognized as a potential risk factor in the development of AK and nonmelanoma skin cancers. In 2011, the FDA stated that sunscreen labels must emphasize protection against both UVA and UVB radiation by "broad-spectrum protection"; therefore, oxybenzone, sulisobenzone, avobenzone, and/or PABA (p-aminobenzoic acid) or a PABA ester if people are sensitive to PABA must be an ingredient in these broad-spectrum SPFs, as they are UVA-protective chemicals. Chemical-free alternatives are known as physical blockers or mineral

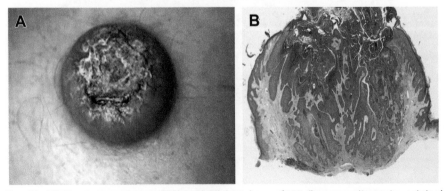

Fig. 15. (A) Keratoancanthoma (KA) and (B) histology of KA (hematoxylin-eosin, original magnification ×40). (*From* Rapini RP. Practical dermatopathology. Philadelphia: Elsevier Mosby; 2005; with permission.)

Box 5
High-risk SCC

- Diameter greater than 2 cm
- Depth greater than 4 mm and Clark level IV or V
- Tumor involvement of bone, muscle, nerve
- Location on ear, lip
- Tumor arising in a scar
- Borders grade 3 or 4
- Patient immunosuppression
- Absence of inflammatory infiltrate

Data from Wolff K, Goldsmith LA, Katz SI, et al, editors. Fitzpatrick's dermatology in general medicine. 7th edition. New York: McGraw-Hill; 2008. p. 1038–9.

---

sunscreens that can reflect UVA and UVB radiation. Titanium dioxide and zinc oxide are the 2 main ingredients in such sunscreens and are recommended to be started in children as young as 6 months of age. Protection at an early age will greatly reduce the incidence of AK or nonmelanoma skin cancers. The best protection is shelter (shade) and avoidance of direct sun exposure during the peak hours of the day (10 AM–4 PM), and protective clothing, along with the reapplication of SPF every 2 hours,

---

Box 6
SCC surgical and nonsurgical treatment modalities

Surgical

Surgery (excisional surgery, Mohs, ED&C, cryosurgery): This is the best management and recommended treatment modality.

Excisional Surgery: Recommend margins 4 mm for low-risk lesions or SCC with depth less than 2 mm. *Cure rate*: 92%.

Mohs Micrographic Surgery: Choice for minimal destruction of tissue and increased tissue preservation (nose, lip, eyelid, ear, nail bed, genitalia), poorly defined clinical margins or deeply infiltrative tumors, involvement of underlying structures (nerve, bone, muscle), scarred lesions, history or radiation sites, lesions with high recurrence rates (lips), or immunosuppressed patients. Depth greater than 6 mm or diameter greater than 1 cm. *Cure rate*: Highest at 94% to 99%.

ED&C: Treatment for low-risk SCC on the trunk and extremities. Process is repeated several times to maximize the probability of complete tumor extirpation.[30] Margin evaluation is uncertain. *Cure rate*: For small primary in situ SCC may be as high as 96%.[30]

Cryosurgery: Generally for special circumstances and only for in situ SCC.

Nonsurgical

RT: Cure rate 85% to 95% and limited to tumors difficult to treat by surgery or special circumstances (ie, elderly patients).

Pharmacologic Therapy: Topical chemotherapies, such as topical cytostatic agents (5-FU) or immunomodulators (Imiquimod), are not FDA approved for treatment of in situ or invasive SCC, but successful treatment has been reported with SCC in situ.

Data from Wolff K, Goldsmith LA, Katz SI, et al, editors. Fitzpatrick's dermatology in general medicine. 7th edition. New York: McGraw-Hill; 2008. p. 1038–9.

because the body metabolizes the SPF within that time or may be removed by swimming or sweating.

SUMMARY & DISCUSSION

Often the skin in sun-exposed areas reveals the telltale signs of sun damage including wrinkles, pigment changes, ephelides, solar lentigines, loss of elasticity, and broken blood vessels. Individuals at risk of developing AK, BCC, and SCC are those with a history of high-risk factors such as UV radiation exposure, genetic makeup, personal or family history, organ transplant recipients, and those with low immune systems and should be monitored closely. Nonetheless, the practitioner is responsible for educating the patient and the public on the prevention of AK and nonmelanoma skin cancers to decrease the chance of becoming a statistic. By encouraging monthly self-examinations as well as complete skin examinations that include the mucosal surfaces on a regular basis, this can help diagnose the AK or nonmelanoma skin cancer early, which can be easily treated. The prognosis is excellent if detected early and for cases that have not metastasized. This summary provides a general review of available treatment options for the management of AK, BCC, and SCC as well as allowing the clinician to use this information as a guideline by applying these therapies on a case-by-case basis to reach the best therapeutic outcomes needed in each individual with a diagnosis of AK, BCC, and/or SCC.

REFERENCES

1. Tierney LM, McPhee SJ, Papadakis MA. Current medical diagnosis and treatment. Prevention of cancer, lifestyle modifications. Chapter 4. Lange Medical Publications; 1999. p. 75.
2. Hoerster KD, Garrow RL, Mayer JA, et al. Density of indoor tanning facilities in 116 large US cities. Am J Prev Med 2009;36:243–6.
3. Fitzpatrick JE, Morelli JG. Dermatology secrets in color. VII. malignant tumors of the skin. Chapter 44. 3rd edition. Elsevier Health Sciences; 2006. p. 361–9.
4. Tung R, Vidimos A. Nonmelanoma skin cancer. The Cleveland Clinic Foundation. Cleveland Clinic Center for Continuing Education; 2009. p. 200–2015. Available at: http://clevelandclinicmeded.com/medicalpubs/diseasemanagement/dermatology/nonmelanoma-skin-cancer/#top.
5. DermNet NZ. Facts about the skin from New Zealand trust. The structure of normal skin. Available at: http://www.dermnetnz.org/pathology/skin-structure.html. Accessed July 5, 2015.
6. American Academy of Dermatology. Available at: www.aad.org.
7. Criscione VD, Weinstock MA, Naylor MF, et al. Actinic keratoses natural history and risk of malignant transformation in the Veterans Affairs Tropical Tretinoin Chemoprevention Trial. Cancer 2009;115:2523–30.
8. Berman B. Advances in Actinic Keratosis Treatments. SDPA Summer Conference. Las Vegas (NV), June 7, 2015.
9. Medscape reference, drugs, diseases & procedures: actinic keratosis: practice essentials, background, pathophysiology. Available at: http://emedicine.medscape.com/article/1099775-overview#showall.
10. Del Rosso J, Kircik L, Brian B. Comprehensive management of actinic keratosis. Practical integration of available therapies with a review of a newer treatment approach. J Clin Aesthet Dermatol 2014;7(9 Suppl S2–S12):S2–12.

11. Medscape reference, drugs, diseases & procedures: basal cell carcinoma: practice essentials, background, pathophysiology. Available at: http://emedicine. medscape.com/article/276624.
12. Brown University. Stem cell classification. Available at: http://www.biomed.brown.edu/ Courses/Bl108/Bl108_2002_Groups/pancstems/stemcell/stemcellsclassversatility.htm.
13. Spencer JM, Hazan C, Hsiung SH, et al. Therapeutic decision making in the therapy of actinic keratosis. J Drugs Dermatol 2005;4(3):296–301 [Medline].
14. Tutrone WD, Saini R, Caglar S, et al. Crespo. Topical therapy of actinic keratosis, I: 5-fluorouracil and imiquimod. Cutis 2003;71(5):365–70 [Medline].
15. Tutrone WD, Saini R, Caglar S, et al. Crespo. Topical therapy of actinic keratosis, II: diclofenac, colchicine, and retinoids. Cutis 2003;71(5):373–9 [Medline].
16. Sobrero A, Guglielmi A, Grossi F, et al. Mechanism of action of fluoropyrimidines: relevance to the new developments in colorectal cancer chemotherapy. Semin Oncol 2000;27(5 Suppl 10):72–7.
17. Fluorouracil cream, FDA package insert of fluorouracil cream USP, 0.5% (Microsphere).
18. Kaur RR, Alikhan A, Maibach HI. Comparison of topical 5-fluorouracil formulations in actinic keratosis treatment. J Dermatolog Treat 2010;21(5):267–71.
19. Jorizzo J, Weiss J, Vamvakias G. One-week treatment with 0.5% fluorouracil cream prior to cryosurgery in patients with actinic keratosis: a double-blind, vehicle-controlled, long-term study. J Drugs Dermatol 2006;5(2):133–9 [Medline].
20. Solaraze gel, FDA package insert of diclogenac sodium gel 3%.
21. Berlin JM, Rigel DS. Diclogenac sodium 3% gel in the treatment of actinic keratosis postcryosurgery. J Drugs Dermatol 2008;7(7):669–73 [Medline].
22. Imiquimod cream. FDA package insert of imiquimod cream 2.5%, 3.75%, 5%.
23. Rosen RH, Gupta AK, Tyring SK. Dual mechanism of action of ingenol mebutate gel for topical treatment of actinic keratosis: rapid lesion necrosis followed by lesion-specific immune response. J Am Acad Dermatol 2012;66(3):486–93 [Medline].
24. Skin Cancer Foundation. Skin cancer facts. 2015. Available at: http://www. skincancer.org.
25. American Cancer Society. Cancer facts & figures. 2015.Available at: http://www. cancer.org.
26. Wolff K. Fitzpatrick's dermatology in general medicine, vol. 1. Chapter 115. 7th edition. McGraw-Hill Professional; 2006. p. 1038–9.
27. Buljan M, Bulat V, Situm M, et al. Variations in clinical presentation of basal cell carcinoma. Acta Clin Croat 2008;47(1):25–30.
28. Dinehart SM. What's new and what's neat in the treatment of non-melanoma skin cancer. Lecture; SDPA Summer Conference. Las Vegas (NV), June 3–7, 2015.
29. Barry J, Oon SF, Watson R, et al. The management of basal cell carcinomas. Ir Med J 2006;99(6):179–81 [Medline].
30. Medscape reference, drugs, diseases, & procedures: cutaneous squamous cell carcinoma: practice essentials, background, pathophysiology. Available at: http://emedicince.medscape.com/article/1965430.
31. Sekulic A, Migden MR, Oro AE, et al. Efficacy and safety of vismodegib in advanced basal-cell carcinoma. N Engl J Med 2012;366(23):2171–9.

An Overview of Rosacea and Its Challenges

 CrossMark

Heather Adams, MPAS, PA-C[a],*, Chelsey Coven, MPAS, PA-C[b],
Kristen M. Grippe, MPAS, PA-C[c]

KEYWORDS

- Rosacea • *Demodex* • Rosacea subtypes • Chronic dermatologic condition
- Public misconceptions • Dermatology Life Quality Index
- Primary and secondary features • Holistic health care approach

KEY POINTS

- Rosacea is a chronic dermatologic condition consisting of various subtypes and degrees of severity.
- The diagnosis of rosacea can be challenging and is often shrouded with misconceptions.
- Several theories regarding the etiology of rosacea exist; the *Demodex* mite is thought to play a significant role in the disorder.
- Rosacea is associated with specific primary and secondary clinical features contributing to the clinical nature of this diagnosis.
- Various treatment options exist allowing for a holistic approach to management of rosacea. Clinician understanding and patient education are essential for compliance and successful treatment.

INTRODUCTION

Rosacea is a common, chronic, relapsing inflammatory skin condition consisting of various subtypes and degrees of severity. It is characterized by flushing, persistent erythema, telangiectasia, papules, and pustules; it primarily affects the convex areas of the face including the nose, cheeks, chin, forehead, glabella, and eyes.[1,2] The condition affects more than 14 million people and is more common in Celtic, northern European, and fair-skinned patients; however, it may be seen in all ethnicities and skin types.[1–4] It tends to affect women between 30 and 50 years of age, but it can affect both men and women of all ages with men more likely to develop severe symptoms including rhinophyma.[1,4]

Disclosure Statement: None of the above names authors have any financial affiliates, commercial or financial conflicts of interest, or sources of funding to disclose.
[a] Gannon University, 109 University Sq, Erie, PA 16541, USA; [b] 377 Porterfield Hill Road, Cowansville, PA 16218, USA; [c] Gannon University, 109 University Sq, Erie, PA 16541, USA
* Corresponding author.
E-mail address: adams051@gannon.edu

Physician Assist Clin 1 (2016) 255–264
http://dx.doi.org/10.1016/j.cpha.2015.12.002
physicianassistant.theclinics.com
2405-7991/16/$ – see front matter © 2016 Elsevier Inc. All rights reserved.

There are a myriad of challenges associated with the diagnosis and treatment of rosacea. The etiology of rosacea is not understood fully and it is largely a clinical diagnosis, lending to potential misdiagnosis or mistreatment because it can mimic other dermatologic conditions such as acne vulgaris or seborrheic dermatitis. Additionally, rosacea is often shrouded by misconceptions, which can lead to poor care and compliance and ultimately negative outcomes for the patient.[2,5] A common misconception is that rosacea is caused by alcoholism owing to a flushed appearance and bloodshot eyes, thus leading to potential undue distress, wrongful judgment, and social exclusion for these patients.[1,2,5] Therefore, it is necessary for health care providers to dispel misconceptions and to provide accurate and current resources for their patients (**Table 1**).[2–4] Rosacea can be a distressing condition that may have negative psychosocial impacts related to facial disfigurement, resulting in more damage to a patient's self-image than to the patient's skin. A thorough discussion of rosacea is necessary to clarify these challenges and aid in appropriate diagnosis and treatment of this condition.

ETIOLOGY

The etiology of rosacea is not understood fully, but many theories exist and studies are underway. Some proposed causes of rosacea include damage to dermal connective tissue often owing to ultraviolet radiation, abnormal vascular reactivity, abnormal inflammatory response, abnormal profibrotic mediator factor XIII in phymatous rosacea, and overpopulation of *Demodex* mites.[1–3,5–8]

Taking a closer look at the role of the innate immune system highlights the likelihood that the etiology of rosacea is multifactorial. The innate immune system is programmed to respond to the environmental factors that have been implicated in the development of rosacea, namely, exposure to ultraviolet light, damage to dermal connective tissue, and microbes such as *Demodex* mites.[8] Increased susceptibility of the skin to these environmental factors in the form of an increased immune response supports the multifactorial theory for the etiology of rosacea.[8] Vascular hyperactivity is closely associated with flushing, a symptom that is commonly seen in rosacea. This can also be the result of an overactive innate immunity.[8]

Of specific interest in this article is the microbe *Demodex*, which has been the source of much discussion regarding the etiology of rosacea. *Demodex* is an obligate human ectoparasitic mite that resides in or adjacent to the pilosebaceous unit where the mite ingests sebum.[5] There are more than 60 *Demodex* species, 2 of which are typically found on humans, *Demodex folliculorum* and *D brevisare*, which are collectively referred to as *Demodex* when discussing the role of these mites in the development and natural history of rosacea. *Demodex* is commonly found on the balding scalp, neck, ears, and face, including the cheeks, nose, chin, forehead, temples, eye lashes, and eyebrows.

Table 1 Resources for information on rosacea	
Name of Resources	**Website Link to Resource**
National Institute of Arthritis and Musculoskeletal and Skin Diseases	www.niams.nih.gov/
American Academy of Dermatology	www.aad.org/
National Rosacea Society	www.rosacea.org/

Data from Refs.[2–4]

Demodex infestation is common with a prevalence varying between 23% to 100% in healthy adults; however, infestation typically remains asymptomatic.[5] The Dermatopathology Service of Mexico's General Hospital conducted a study in which skin biopsies of patients with clinically diagnosed rosacea were compared with skin biopsies of a control group consisting of patient who were not diagnosed with rosacea.[6] The study found that *D folliculorum* was present in 80% of rosacea biopsies and 30% of control biopsies, and the mean infestation density of *D folliculorum* was higher in the rosacea biopsies than in the control biopsies.[6] *Demodex* seems to play an important role in the pathophysiology of *Demodex*-type rosacea. Some proposed mechanisms include direct damage to the follicular epithelia, generation of foreign body reactions, induction of host hypersensitivity, and action as a vector for bacteria. *Demodex* may damage the follicular epithelia by increased mite density, or by obstruction of the hair follicle or sebaceous duct.[5,6]

CLINICAL PRESENTATION AND DIAGNOSIS

The recognition of rosacea by its primary and secondary features is key to making an accurate diagnosis and aiding in the development of an appropriate treatment plan. The primary features of rosacea include nontransient erythema, which is the most common sign, and presents as persistent erythema that does not wax or wane with trigger exposure. Transient erythema may occur in the form of blushing or flushing, telangiectasia, papules, and pustules.[1,4] Secondary features may either coexist with primary features or exist independently. Secondary features include burning or stinging sensations, plaques, dry appearance, edema, ocular manifestations, rosacea present at other nonfacial sites, and phymatous changes.[1,4] To diagnosis rosacea, 1 or more of the primary features must be present in the central distribution of the face. A committee of experts of the National Rosacea Society developed a standard classification system to aid health care providers in the diagnosis and treatment of rosacea, including primary and secondary features of the various subtypes (**Table 2**).

Facial appearance plays a large role in self-perception, self-esteem, and interaction with others.[2,4,5] Consequently, the condition may cause embarrassment, insecurity, and loss of confidence. As a result, rosacea patients may develop depression, social anxiety or phobia, or body dysmorphic disorder.[2,5] The National Rosacea Society conducted a patient survey in 2000 showing that 75% and 70% of rosacea patients experienced low self-esteem and embarrassment, respectively.[4] The effects of rosacea drastically interfere with patients' activities of daily living, which ultimately decreases their quality of life.[1,5] It is paramount that health care providers assess their patients' quality of life using a quick, simple assessment tool, such as the Dermatology Life Quality Index. The Dermatology Life Quality Index consists of 10 questions that relate to the ways in which skin conditions impact the lives of patients. Available at: www.cardiff.ac.uk/dermatology/.[1,2,5]

A diagnosis of rosacea is made largely through the clinical assessment and evaluation of symptomatology, and those symptoms may be further grouped into 4 subtypes. The 4 subtypes of rosacea are erythematotelangiectactic, papulopustular, phymatous, and ocular. Patients may manifest with 1 subtype, multiple subtypes, or patients may progress through the subtypes.[2,4] Additionally, the different types of rosacea can mimic other skin conditions in their clinical presentation, increasing the potential for misdiagnosis. It is essential to differentiate other skin disorders, such as acne vulgaris, lupus erythematosus, perioral dermatitis, seborrheic dermatitis, and topical steroid misuse, from rosacea. Papulopustular rosacea is commonly mistaken for acne vulgaris; however, acne vulgaris may present with comedones

Table 2
Primary and secondary features of rosacea

Features	Description
Primary	
Flushing	Transient erythema
Persistent flushing	Nontransient erythema
Papules and Pustules	• Crops of dome-shaped red papules • Pustules may or may not be present • May be nodular • Noncomedonal
Telangiectasia	Dilated vessels
Secondary	
Burning or stinging sensations	With or without scaling or dermatitis
Plaques	• Elevated • Red
Dry appearance	Rough, scaly, dry skin in central distribution of face
Edema	Usually after prolonged flushing or erythema
Ocular manifestations	• Burning • Itching • Bloodshot eyes • Eyelid inflammation • Sties • Corneal damage
Rosacea present at nonfacial sites	• Neck • Scalp • Ears • Back
Phymatous changes	• Patulous follicles • Skin thickening and fibrosis • Bulbous appearance • Most commonly affects the nose (rhinophyma)

Data from Refs.[1-5]

and rosacea lacks comedones. Rosacea may coexist with other skin disorders, such as acne vulgaris, making diagnosis challenging. Consequently, both a thorough history and clinical examination in a proper facility with good lighting is important to establish the correct diagnosis.[1] The following sections discuss the major subtypes of rosacea in detail.

Erythematotelangiectatic Rosacea

Erythematotelangiectatic rosacea is characterized by the key features of persistent flushing and nontransient central facial erythema. Telangiectasia is common in this subtype; however, it may be absent and is not essential for diagnosis.[1-5] Other symptoms can include burning and stinging sensations, edema of the central face, scaling, and roughness. A patient with this subtype may have minimal or no inflammatory lesions. A sensitivity to topical products is common and may contribute to flushing or erythema.[2-5]

Papulopustular Rosacea

Papulopustular rosacea is defined as persistent facial erythema with transient papules and/or pustules, and typically involves the central face. Perioral, perinasal, and periocular areas may be affected as well.[1–5] This subtype can be seen in combination with erythematotelangiectatic rosacea; therefore, flushing and edema may be present.[2–5] Symptoms may include stinging and burning sensations and sensitivity to facial and topical products.[2,5]

Phymatous Rosacea

Phymatous rosacea occurs in a minority of cases, but it is associated with higher rates of disfigurement secondary to irreversible hypertrophy of affected skin, which can lead to major impacts on patients' psychological health.[1] Signs include thickening of the skin, irregular surface nodularities, and enlargement of facial features. It most commonly affects the nose, giving rise to the bulbous appearance in rhinophyma, but it may involve the forehead, cheeks, ears, and chin.[1–5] Symptoms may include stinging and burning sensations and soreness.[2,5]

Ocular Rosacea

Ocular rosacea is common, affecting up to one-half of patients with rosacea.[1,3] Symptoms involving the eyes include sensation of a foreign body, burning, stinging, dryness, itchiness, photosensitivity, and blurred vision. Blepharitis, conjunctivitis, and periorbital edema may also be present and eyes may seem to be watery or bloodshot.[1–5]

Demodex-type Rosacea

Demodex-type rosacea may be seen in patients who have high densities of *Demodex* mites. This type of rosacea is not currently seen as a fifth subtype, but rather as a rosacea-like demodicidosis or dry type of rosacea. *Demodex*-type rosacea is characterized by dryness, follicular scaling, superficial vesicles, and pustules.[5] For diagnosis of *Demodex*-type rosacea, health care providers have to confirm the presence of *Demodex*. Assessment methods for *Demodex* include skin surface biopsy with cyanoacylic adhesion and microscopy assessment using adhesive bands, skin scrapings, skin impressions, expressed follicular contents, comedone extractions, hair epilations, and punch biopsies. However, with the prevalence of *Demodex* infection approaching 100% in the general population, the mere presence of *Demodex* does not indicate pathogenesis.[7] The density of the mite infestation is more important, with greater than 5 mites per follicle serving as the diagnostic criteria.[5]

TREATMENT

The goals of therapy are to control the natural history of rosacea, prevent complications, and improve quality of life. Treatments should be selected based on the type of rosacea, the severity of clinical features, patient history, patient quality of life, and patient preference.[3] All patients should follow general measures specific to either common forms of rosacea or *Demodex*-type rosacea (**Box 1**).[2] The majority of patients respond well to treatments, but improvement is often gradual and it can take 3 months or more to see results. Patients should be made aware of this along with realistic expectations of treatment to help improve patient compliance.[1,2,5]

Trigger Avoidance

To obtain the best results from treatment, a rosacea patient should be educated about possible triggers that may worsen the condition as well as the importance of avoiding these triggers.[1,4] Triggers include but are not limited to ultraviolet radiation, extremes of temperature, strong winds, exercise, alcohol, spicy hot foods, hot drinks, red wine,

---

Box 1
General measures in the management of rosacea and *Demodex*-type rosacea

Rosacea

Keep face cool

Exercise in air conditioning

Avoid overheating, warm rooms, and hot baths and showers

Cover face on windy or cold days

Avoid washing with soap and astringent cleaners or wipes

Wash face gently with emollient washes and avoid overwashing and scrubbing

Avoid oil-based facial products and wipes by using aqueous-based products

Avoid products containing alcohol, hazel, menthol, peppermint, and clove oil

Moisturize daily and often in dry climate and warm weather and to soothe stinging and burning

Avoid food and beverage triggers such as alcohol and hot, spicy foods

Wear sun protection factor 30 sunscreen with titanium dioxide or zinc oxide all year round

Control and manage stress and emotions in healthy behaviors

Quit smoking

Follow-up with health care provider on a regular basis

Demodex-Type Rosacea

Cleanse face twice daily with nonsoap cleanser

Avoid oil-based cleansers and greasy makeup

Exfoliate periodically to remove dead skin cells

Data from Refs.[1-5]

---

topical steroids, stress, and numerous skin care products, especially those containing alcohol.[1,2,5] Furthermore, stressful emotions such as anger, anxiety, and frustration can cause flares, so it is important to educate patients on stress and emotion management techniques such as deep breathing exercises, visualization techniques, yoga, talk therapy, meditation, and support groups.[3] Patients may be encouraged to keep a food or activity diary to help isolate potential triggers.[1]

Topical Agents

Topical agents generally serve as first-line therapy for the erythematotelangiectic or papulopustular subtypes as long as symptoms are only of mild to moderate severity. Topical agents can be used in acute flares, but are most effective for the maintenance of remission.[1,3,5] First-line topical agents are metronidazole, azelaic acid, and sulfacetamide.[3,4] Metronidazole is available in a 0.75% preparation as a gel, cream, or lotion and a 1% preparation is available in a gel (MetroGel 1%) or cream (Noritate). Azelaic acid is available in a 20% cream (Azelex) and a 15% gel (Finacea). The most common side effects of these topical agents may include dryness, inflammation, or stinging.[1,4] Selection of preparations is based on both the patient's skin type and area of treatment; for example, creams are preferred for moist areas and lotions are preferred on the scalp.[4,9] Second-tier agents are topical erythromycin (Akne-Mycin) and clindamycin phosphate 1% (Cleocin T, Clindagel, ClindaMax).[3,4] Overall, these first- and second-tier topical agents are used to decrease erythema and inflammatory lesions. Compared with oral therapies, topical agents have fewer side effects and tolerability issues. However, their effects are slower in onset, resulting in a longer period of time before desired results are achieved.[3]

Other topical agents that have been studied but are not considered first line include tacrolimus, pimecrolimus, and topical retinoids such as adapalene or tretinoin. Both tacrolimus and pimecrolimus may reduce inflammation and itching, whereas tretinoin may reduce inflammation and lesions.[3] Anti-*Demodex* treatments such as topical ivermectin (Soolantra), permethrin cream, crotamiton cream, and lindane have been studied but are not mainstream.[3,5,10] These creams are antiparasitics and are used to kill *Demodex* in *Demodex*-type rosacea. A key feature of *Demodex*-type rosacea is its complete resolution with the use of antiparasitics.[5,7,10]

Oral Therapies and Side Effects

Oral therapies are reserved for moderate to severe cases of papulopustular and ocular forms of rosacea. Common first-line oral therapies are used to reduce inflammation, papules, and pustules; these include tetracycline, doxycycline, and minocycline (**Table 3**).[3,4] When used to treat rosacea these antibiotics serve as antiinflammatory agents rather than antimicrobial agents. This allows for the utilization of submicrobial doses of these antibiotics to help with decreasing side effects as well as antibiotic resistance.[11] Common side effects of doxycycline include heartburn, nausea, vomiting, diarrhea, and ultraviolet photosensitivity. Minocycline may cause headache, dizziness, arthralgias, myalgias, or skin and/or gingival discolorations that presents as slate gray patches that are commonly mistaken for persistent bruises. Oral medications should be discontinued if any of these symptoms occur, or if other hypersensitivity reactions such as urticaria develop. It is important to counsel pregnant patients that tetracyclines are contraindicated in the second and third trimesters owing to various fetal

Table 3
First-line oral therapies used in treatment of rosacea

Oral Antibiotic	Dose	Common Side Effect Profile
Tetracycline	500 mg BID	Nausea Vomiting Diarrhea Epigastric discomfort
Doxycycline	100 mg BID	Photosensitivity Nausea Diarrhea

Modified-released
    preparation
	20 mg BID or	Fewer GI side effects than
		    antimicrobial doxycycline 100 mg BID

Doxycycline
    (subantimicrobial)
	40 mg once daily	Less antibiotic resistance than
		    antimicrobial doxycycline

Minocycline	100 mg BID	Nausea Vomiting Diarrhea Epigastric discomfort Vertigo Hyperpigmentation Lupus-like syndrome

Abbreviations: BID, twice a day; GI, gastrointestinal.
Data from Refs.[1,3–5,11]

and maternal adverse effects.[12] Other oral therapies include metronidazole, erythromycin, trimethoprim/sulfamethoxazole, and clarithromycin.[1,3–5] Oral therapies have better success rates with preventing papules and pustules than topical agents but are associated with more adverse side effects. Patients can expect to see about a 50% decrease in inflammatory lesions after 3 months of use, and increased clearance is usually seen as treatment continues. However, there is a concern about antibiotic resistance from long-term use.[3,5]

For more severe cases of rosacea that do not respond to topical or other oral therapies, oral isotretinoin may be prescribed. Isotretinoin improves the symptoms of severe rosacea, including papules, pustules, and rhinopyma.[1,2,4] Dosages as low as 10 mg/d have been associated with successful treatment, but common dosages average 40 to 80 mg/d in divided doses. Therapy continues for approximately 5 months or until a total of 120 to 150 mg/kg is consumed. Common side effects of isotretinoin include skin and mucosal dryness, with cheilits occurring in 90% of cases, epistaxis, fatigue, arthralgias, and myalgias. Blood tests should be performed monthly to evaluate for anemia, liver enzymes, and lipid levels as triglycerides commonly become temporarily elevated. Women of child-bearing potential are required to have a monthly serum or urine pregnancy test. The most significant side effect is severe teratogenicity that consists of a recognizable pattern of multiple fetal defects, making this medication contraindicated in pregnancy.[12] Patients on isotretinoin must register with the iPledge system, an program approved by the US Food and Drug Administration that is designed to help avoid the potentially devastating effects of isotretinoin on a fetus.[1,4] Within this program, isotretinoin prescribers, patients, and pharmacists are required to follow certain rules and regulations, including prescriber and pharmacist certification, documentation of pregnancy testing results, and patient agreement to use contraception or remain abstinent.[13]

In the case of severe rosacea that is unresponsive to topical and oral therapies, complicated by phymatous changes, or has ocular involvement, the patient should be referred to a consultant dermatologist, plastic surgeon, or ophthalmologist.

Interventional Therapy

Laser therapies are effective in the reduction of erythema and telangiectasia of rosacea.[2–4] Examples of lasers used in the treatment of rosacea are pulsed dye and intense pulsed light lasers (IPL), both of which are used to decrease the red appearance of the skin.[4,14]

The basic concept of IPL therapy consists of the absorption of photons by target structures within the skin known as chromophores. This results in the transfer of energy in the form of heat leading to photothermolysis and destruction of the target structures.[14] A clinical study conducted by Piccolo and colleagues[14] used IPL and demonstrated that IPL improves rosacea through the ablation of abnormal vessels, the remodeling of collagen, and the reduction of inflammation. The study concluded that rosacea patients required 2 to 5 sessions 20 to 30 days apart for significant results. Moderate reductions in vessel number and size and in papules were observed after the second session with significant reduction in vessel number and size and the complete disappearance of papules after the fourth session. Complete clearance was observed in 70% of patients at 12 months with the remaining 30% of patients requiring treatment for a recurrence of the papulopustular component.[14]

Telangiectasia may also be treated with fine-point electrodessication.[4] Furthermore, rhinophyma may be effectively treated with laser ablation, as well as with dermabrasion, surgical correction, or razor or scalpel remodeling for debulking.[2,4]

Alternative Treatments and Cosmetics

There are a number of homeopathic therapies that may be of benefit for rosacea patients; however, clinical trials for these therapies are limited and some natural therapies may have adverse side effects, especially when combined with prescription medications. Natural therapies include chrysanthellum indicum and licorice cream to reduce redness, green tea to reduce erythematous bumps and pustules, niacinamine to improve the skin barrier and reduce redness, aloe to reduce irritation, and chamomile to reduce inflammation. Avoidance of foods known to cause inflammation, such as caffeine, alcoholic beverages, "fast foods," high-fat meats, processed foods, high-sugar foods, tomatoes, candy (with the exception of dark chocolate), gluten additives, and refined carbohydrates can be important for prevention of symptoms.[3] Patients can also add foods that are antiinflammatory in nature, such as B vitamins, ginger, tumeric, omega 3 fatty acids, and olive oil.[3]

Finally, camouflage cosmetics are a good option for rosacea patients who wish to disguise persistent redness or cover up lesions. Many of these cosmetics use a base with a green tint to conceal unwanted erythema and abnormalities.[1–3]

Patient Education

Patient education is an essential component of the overall care of patients with rosacea; patients who understand their diagnosis and treatment(s) are more likely to experience positive outcomes. A Finacea Patient Survey conducted by the National Rosacea Society in 2000 reported that 87% of rosacea patients were more compliant with therapy after learning about their condition.[3] Although topical and oral therapies are effective, more than 60% of patients on both topical and oral therapy relapse within 6 months, illustrating the importance of follow-up care. Patients should follow-up in 4 weeks after initiation of a therapy to assess the progress and tolerability of the treatment. After desired control is achieved, patients can follow-up every 3 to 6 months for reevaluation. At follow-up visits, health care providers should assess current treatment success and consider alternative therapies as needed, offer patient education, and provide avenues for patient support.[5]

SUMMARY

Rosacea is a chronic condition composed of various subtypes and a spectrum of symptom severity. Accurate and specific diagnosis, keeping in mind the possibility of Demodex-type rosacea, can allow for effective treatment and control via a combination of topical and/or oral medications, avoidance of triggers, patient education, exploration of interventional and alternative therapies, and proper follow-up care.[5] It is important for health care providers to dispel misconceptions and to assess patients' quality of life because rosacea can have a negative impact on a person's psychosocial health.[2,5] In conclusion, when health care providers possess a comprehensive knowledge of rosacea as a medical condition as well as a thorough understanding of the diagnostic criteria and various treatment options, they will be able to contribute to the optimal holistic health care of their patients with this chronic dermatologic condition.[5]

REFERENCES

1. Oliver P, Courtenay M. The red face: recognising and managing rosacea. Prim Health Care 2010;20(3):16–20. Available at: http://web.a.ebscohost.com.ezproxy.gannon. edu/ehost/pdfviewer/pdfviewer   ?sid=2f7ac470-f681-4bd1-a652-1719f10f75ac% 40sessionmgr4005&vid=&hid= 4109. Accessed October 18, 2014.

2. Van Onselen J. Rosacea: symptoms and support. Br J Nurs 2012;21(21):1252–5. Available at: http://web.b.ebscohost.com.ezproxy.gannon.edu/ehost/pdfviewer/pdfviewer?sid=17f4d358-a54f-4135-b900-59b14e9afd57%40sessionmgr113&vid=7&hid=109. Accessed October 18, 2014.

3. Barton ML. Rosacea management- why it matters: nursing implications and patient education. Dermatol Nurs 2008;20(6):10–4. Available at: http://search.proquest.com.ezproxy.gannon.edu/docview/224823509/fulltextPDF/D6CBEE8023EB428APQ/1?accountid=36086. Accessed October 18, 2014.

4. Hoag S, Raspa RF. Help for the patient with rosacea. Patient Care 2007;41:9–12. Available at: http://web.a.ebscohost.com.ezproxy.gannon.edu/ehost/pdfviewer/pdfviewer?sid=2f7ac470-f681-4bd1-a652-1719f10f75ac%40sessionmgr4005&vid=7&hid=4109. Accessed October 18, 2014.

5. Van Onselen J. Prescribing for mild-to-moderate rosacea. NursePrescribing 2012;10(1):25–31. Available at: http://web.b.ebscohost.com.ezproxy.gannon.edu/ehost/pdfviewer/pdfviewer?sid=17f4d358-a54f-4135-b900-59b14e9afd57%40sessionmgr113&vid=10&hid=109. Accessed October 18, 2014.

6. Ríos-Yuil JM, Mercadillo-Perez P. Evaluation of Demodex folliculorum as a risk factor for the diagnosis of rosacea in skin biopsies. Mexico's General Hospital (1975-2010). Indian J Dermatol 2013;58(2):157. Available at: http://search.proquest.com.ezproxy.gannon.edu/docview/1323496604/fulltextPDF/B43304DB2715498APQ/1?accountid=36086. Accessed October 18, 2014.

7. Rather PA, Hassan I. Human Demodex mite: the versatile mite of dermatological importance. Indian J Dermatol 2014;59(1):60–6. Available at: http://search.proquest.com.ezproxy.gannon.edu/docview/1477233274/fulltextPDF/FCF0587CED6446BCPQ/2?accountid=36086. Accessed October 18, 2014.

8. Yamasaki K, Gallo RL. The molecular pathology of rosacea. J Dermatol Sci 2009; 55(2):77–81. Available at: www.ncbi.nlm.nih.gov/pmc/articles/PMC2745268/. Accessed June 4, 2015.

9. Topical treatments. British Journal Of Community Nursing [serial online] 2014;38–83. 46p. Available at: CINAHL with Full Text, Ipswich, MA. Accessed January 8, 2016.

10. Kligman AM, Christensen MS. Demodex folliculorum: requirements for understanding its role in human skin disease. J Invest Dermatol 2011;131(1):8–10. Available at: http://search.proquest.com.ezproxy.gannon.edu/docview/817450872/fulltextPDF/54DD391DA1924CA8PQ/1?accountid=36086. Accessed October 18, 2014.

11. Rosen T. Antibiotic resistance: an editorial review with recommendations. J Drugs Dermatol 2011;10:724–33.

12. Briggs GG, Freeman RK, Sumner JF. Drugs in pregnancy and lactation. 10th edition. New York: Lippincott Williams & Wilkins; 2015. p. 745–7, 1339–1341.

13. iPledge information. U.S. food and drug administration web site. 2010. Available at: www.fda.gov/Drugs/DrugSafety/PostmarketDrugSafetyInformationforPatientsandProviders/ucm094307.htm. Accessed January 4, 2015.

14. Piccolo D, Di Marcantonio D, Crisman G, et al. Unconventional use of intense pulsed light. Biomed Res Int 2014;2014:618206. Available at: http://search.proquest.com.ezproxy.gannon.edu/docview/1564617084/fulltextPDF/FEC0BB59D0A742FCPQ/1?accountid=36086. Accessed October 18, 2014.

Cutis Marmorata Telangiectatica Congenita

Diagnostic Considerations and Challenges of This Multifocal Disorder

Eileen Cheever, MPAS, PA-C*

KEYWORDS

- Cutis marmorata telangiectatica congenita • Reticulate erythema • Ulceration
- Atrophy • Asymmetry

KEY POINTS

- Cutis marmorata telangiectatica congenita (CMTC) is a condition of unknown cause characterized by reticulate erythema, telangiectasia, and phlebectasia.
- Multiple causes have been hypothesized including increased maternal serum beta human chorionic gonadotropin, the Happle lethal gene hypothesis, autosomal dominance, high levels of serum free copper, teratogens, fetal ascites, lack of mesodermic vessel development, and peripheral neural dysfunction.
- Extracutaneous findings are common with CMTC, with limb asymmetry being the most frequently diagnosed finding.
- Valid diagnostic criteria are not yet available, but current suggested criteria may help guide the diagnosis.
- Prognosis is generally good in CMTC, but all children should have multidisciplinary follow-up annually during the first 3 years of life to evaluate for new-onset extracutaneous findings.

INTRODUCTION

Cutis marmorata telangiectatica congenita (CMTC) is a cutaneous congenital vascular anomaly of unknown cause, consisting of persistent cutis marmorata, phlebectasia, and telangiectasia.[1] Ulceration and atrophy of the skin have also been associated with this condition. Van Lohuizen first described the condition in 1922, and he noted reticulate erythema and telangiectasia with skin atrophy and/or ulceration.[2] Cutis is typically localized in a unilateral distribution, with the lower limbs being the most commonly affected. Often, the affected limb shows signs of hypertrophy or

Disclosure: The author has nothing to disclose.
* The Rockoff Dermatology Center, 28 Andover Street, Suite 235, Andover, MA 01810.
E-mail address: emcheever@yahoo.com

Physician Assist Clin 1 (2016) 265–275
http://dx.doi.org/10.1016/j.cpha.2015.12.004
2405-7991/16/$ – see front matter © 2016 Elsevier Inc. All rights reserved.

hypotrophy; body asymmetry is the most common extracutaneous finding in cutis.[3] Involvement of the trunk and face has also been reported.

PREVALENCE

Approximately 300 cases have been reported in the literature.[2] The exact frequency is not known, although early literature in the 1960s cited benign cases without significant complications. It was not until 1970 that Petrozzi and colleagues[4] reported the first case of CMTC in the United States with significant congenital defects. The lesions of CMTC are usually present at birth or shortly after, with some lesions developing later, from 3 months to 2 years of age.[3]

Gender/Race

Gender-related predisposition is not well established. A few published reports infer a female predominance, but the possible gender differences have not been found to be statistically significant.[1] Literature has further suggested a male preponderance for localized versus generalized disease in women, but this has also been refuted in subsequent reports.[5] Race has not been shown to influence the occurrence of CMTC.

RISK FACTORS

The pathogenesis of CMTC is not known, although several causes have been proposed, as noted in **Fig. 1**. Increased maternal beta human chorionic gonadotropin level and fetal ascites have been reported, although a direct relationship has not been shown.[1] The Happle lethal gene theory, in which mosaicism allows the expression of a dominant lethal gene, has also been proposed as a causative factor.[6] An autosomal dominant transmission has also been suggested. Kurczynski[7] reported a case of a 4-year-old female patient with autosomal dominant gene transmission of CMTC via the paternal line, in which the patient's father and paternal grandmother showed early congenital mottling, with apparent improvement by adulthood. Andreev and Pramatarov[8] described 2 adult sisters who both had lesions at birth that did not resolve with adulthood.

Peripheral neural dysfunction and the lack of mesodermic vessel development during the embryonic stage have also been studied without definitive conclusion.[9] High levels of free copper were detected in a 16-month-old boy with CMTC and the investigators suggested that inactivation of copper-dependent alpha1-antitrypsin may contribute to the occurrence of the CMTC phenotype.[10]

Environmental teratogens and viral infections have also been hypothesized, although no specific agent has been pinpointed. A case report published in 1982 detailed 4 patients born between April 1978 and September 1979 with CMTC, all born within a 19.2-km radius of Sydney, Australia.[11] Extensive epidemiologic questioning and work-up were done on both the patients and parents, without a conclusive teratogenic cause identified.

PHYSICAL EXAMINATION

Physical examination remains the standard for diagnosis of CMTC, because histologic findings on biopsy are generally nonspecific. Histologic findings may include dilated capillaries in the deep dermis with dilated venous lakes or veins and swollen endothelial cells.[12] At this time, no laboratory studies exist to confirm or exclude the presence

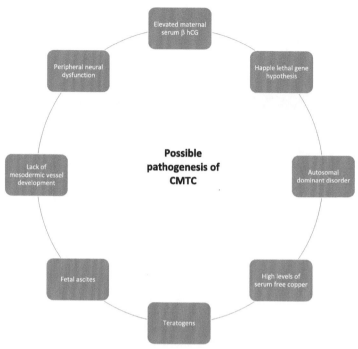

Fig. 1. Possible pathogenesis of CMTC. β hCG, beta human chorionic gonadotropin. (*Data from* Refs.[1,3,6,9–11])

of CMTC. Imaging studies are not indicated unless there are suspected congenital anomalies.[12,13]

Most CMTC presents at birth or shortly after. There have been reports of lesions developing later, from 3 months up to 2 years of age.[3] CMTC typically affects the lower limbs, with upper extremities, trunk, and facial involvement less common.

The cutaneous pattern of the primary lesion is reticulated with a bluish pink discoloration, as shown in **Figs. 2** and **3**. Phlebectasia and telangiectasia are usually present. The areas are frequently serpiginous and depressed, although some lesions are patchy.[14] Some of these lesions have been described as marbled or a having a fishnet appearance.[15] CMTC can be generalized or localized and it is common to see cutaneous atrophy and/or ulceration of the involved skin. The borders of CMTC generally have a sharply demarcated border.[16] Unlike benign cutis marmorata, a common benign physiologic response to cold in infants, CMTC does not respond to warming.[16]

Extracutaneous Findings

Other extracutaneous findings have been reported in 20% to 80% of patients with CMTC.[16] These rates have been criticized because of suspected overlap with other concurrent genetic disorders.[17] The most common extracutaneous finding is body asymmetry, particularly of the limbs. Reported rates of this asymmetry vary, as noted in different studies by Devillers and colleagues[6] (43%), Kienast and Hoeger[2] (33%), and Pehr and Moroz[18] (68%). Glaucoma has also been reported with CMTC, albeit

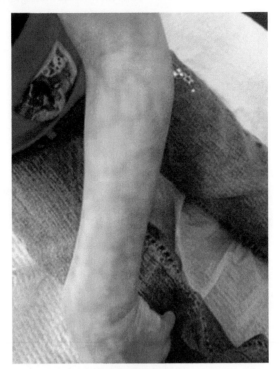

Fig. 2. The reticulate erythema of CMTC, affecting the arm. (*Courtesy of* Eileen Cheever, MPAS, PA-C, Andover, Massachusetts.)

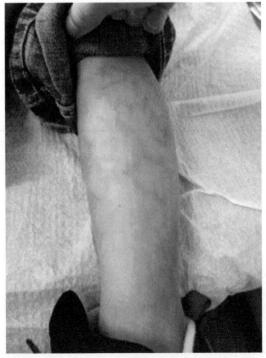

Fig. 3. The reticulate erythema of CMTC, affecting the leg. (*Courtesy of* Eileen Cheever, MPAS, PA-C, Andover, Massachusetts.)

rarely and often in conjunction with other vascular disorders, such as a nevus flammeus involving the affected eye.[4]

Additional extracutaneous findings include, but are not limited to, vascular anomalies, skeletal abnormalities, and neurologic abnormalities, as noted in **Box 1**. Careful and thorough physical examination is warranted in any suspected case of CMTC.

DIAGNOSIS

Accurate and early diagnosis is critical, because children with CMTC are at risk of life-threatening complications and neurologic abnormalities throughout life. Because cutis can present with many cutaneous and extracutaneous findings, as noted earlier, diagnosis can be challenging. Numerous other neurologic and vascular conditions have been associated with CMTC, making the differential diagnoses broad (**Box 2**).

Differential Diagnosis

When working with the differential diagnoses of CMTC, ruling out physiologic cutis marmorata is an appropriate first step. This step can be accomplished by exposing the area to rewarming. If the lesion resolves, physiologic cutis marmorata is generally confirmed and any persisting and/or recurrent physiologic cutis marmorata should have a work-up to rule out medical disorders such as Down syndrome, de Lange syndrome, and homocystinuria. An algorithm for working through the differential diagnoses of CMTC is shown in **Fig. 4**.[3] If the lesion resists rewarming, a more thorough work-up should be done for CMTC, with special attention paid to concurrent vascular lesions, tonometry/visual field assessment, head circumference, musculoskeletal

---

Box 1
Extracutaneous anomalies associated with CMTC

Limb/body asymmetry

Glaucoma

Port-wine stains

Macrocephaly

Developmental delays

Hypotonia

Syndactyly

Hip dysplasia

Clubfoot

Cleft palate

Renal disease

Cardiac malformation

Hypothyroidism

Genitourinary anomalies

Data from De Maio C, Pomero A, Delogu A, et al. Cutis marmorata telangiectatica congenita in a preterm female newborn: case report and review of the literature. Pediatr Med Chir 2014;36(4):161–6; and Levy R, Lam JM. Cutis marmorata telangiectatica congenita: a mimicker of a common disorder. CMAJ 2011;183(4):E249–51.

Box 2
Differential diagnoses of CMTC

Physiologic cutis marmorata

Macrocephaly-CMTC syndrome

Livedo reticularis associated with collagen vascular disease

Klippel-Trénaunay syndrome

Sturge-Weber syndrome

Bockenheimer disease

Nevus flammeus (port-wine stain)

Nevus anemicus

Adams-Oliver syndrome

Divry–van Bogaert syndrome

Data from Schwartz RA, Zalewska A, Onder M, et al. Cutis marmorata telangiectatica congenita. Available at: http://emedicine.medscape.com/article/1086221. Accessed July 7, 2015; and De Maio C, Pomero A, Delogu A et al. Cutis marmorata telangiectatica congenita in a preterm female newborn: case report and review of the literature. Pediatr Med Chir 2014;36(4):161–6.

---

examination (especially limb girth measurement), and neurologic evaluation. Abnormal findings in any of these areas may point to a mimic of CMTC.

Macrocephaly and Cutis Marmorata Telangiectatica Congenita

Nomenclature as it pertains to CMTC has been a source of diagnostic confusion.[19] As such, a noted high frequency of macrocephaly alongside CMTC led to the creation of a distinct diagnostic subtype known as macrocephaly-CMTC (M-CMTC). To date, more than 50 cases have been reported in the literature. This condition was first identified in 1997 by Moore and colleagues,[20] who observed 13 children presenting with CMTC-like cutaneous findings alongside distinct neurologic and connective tissue anomalies. They noted that affected patients frequently present with both CMTC and macrocephaly, as well as developmental delay, neonatal hypotonia, syndactyly, segmental overgrowth, connective tissue defects, and asymmetry.[21]

It has also been proposed that this presentation is a variation of capillary malformation rather than true CMTC. To that point, in 2007, Toriello and Mulliken[14] first proposed renaming M-CMTC to macrocephaly–capillary malformation (M-CM), showing this relationship. They pointed out that the vascular lesions in question are commonly located on the nose and philtrum as well as the limbs and trunk. Furthermore, they pointed out that, unlike CMTC, the lesions never ulcerate and rarely completely resolve.[14] They also noted that size and symmetry of the affected limbs vary greatly between each condition. Because of these apparent differences, they recommended using the term M–CM in these instances to eliminate confusion and misdiagnosis.

As a follow-up to this recommendation, Wright and colleagues[22] published a comprehensive review in 2009 of more than 100 cases, including 12 new cases, that further supports the recommendations of Toriello and Mulliken.[14] This review suggests that the vascular malformations noted in macrocephaly CMTC are actually capillary malformations, of the port-wine or salmon-patch variation. Based on this observation, they support the adaptation of the term M-CM, as proposed by Toriello and Mulliken[14] (**Fig. 5**).

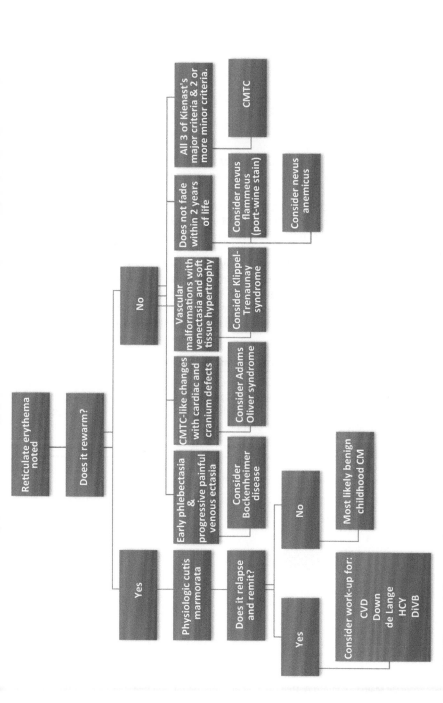

Fig. 4. Potential differential diagnoses for reticulate erythema. CM, cutis marmorata; CVD, collagen vascular disease; DiVB, Divry–van Bogaert syndrome; HCY, homocystinuria. (*Data from* Refs.[1,2,16])

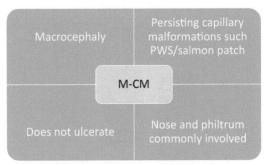

Fig. 5. Components of the proposed term M-CM, as suggested by Toriello and Mulliken[14] and Wright and colleagues.[22] PWS, port-wine stain. (*Data from* Refs.[14,22,23])

In 2011, in an attempt to eliminate the confusion of nomenclature and diagnosis, an article published in the *Journal of European Medical Genetics* proposed a 6-part classification system to categorize vascular malformations and growth disturbances. The investigators not only support the M-CM designation but also classify it into a category known as reticular capillary malformation, type VI.[23] They pointed out that classic CMTC is a separate entity and excluded from this classification system, because of the distinct aplasia cutis (ie, ulceration) that can occur alongside the growth disturbances,[23] which again highlights the importance of a detailed physical examination that includes inspection of skin lesions, head circumference measurement, and screening for developmental delays.

Suggested Diagnostic Criteria for Cutis Marmorata Telangiectatica Congenita

Diagnostic criteria have been proposed for CMTC, but the validity of the proposed criteria has yet to be determined. In 2009, Kienast and Hoeger[2] put forth 3 major criteria and 5 minor criteria for the diagnosis of CMTC (**Box 3**). They suggest that the presence of 3 major and 2 minor criteria is sufficient to indicate CMTC.

Box 3
Kienast and Hoeger[2] recommended diagnostic criteria for CTMC.

Major Criteria

Congenital reticulate erythema

Lack of venectasia

Does not respond to local warming

Minor Criteria

Port-wine stain noted outside of CMTC

Skin ulcer in affected area

Fading erythema within 2 years

Atrophy in affected area

Telangiectasia in affected area

Data from De Maio C, Pomero A, Delogu A, et al. Cutis marmorata telangiectatica congenita in a preterm female newborn: case report and review of the literature. Pediatr Med Chir 2014;36(4):161–6; and Levy R, Lam JM. Cutis marmorata telangiectatica congenita: a mimicker of a common disorder. CMAJ 2011;183(4):E249–51.

MONITORING

Annual multidisciplinary follow-up is recommended for at least 3 years. Visits should include screening for commonly associated anomalies, as described earlier, and monitoring for any possible conditions that can mimic CMTC.[2] Long-term follow-up of CMTC into adolescence and adulthood is sparsely reported, but these reports have detailed a wide range of abnormalities, including persistent reticulate erythema, mental/physical retardation, hypertension, seizures, spinal deformities, and acrocyanosis.[5,8,18,24,25]

PROGNOSIS

The prognosis of CMTC is generally good. Approximately 50% of patients have spontaneous resolution of the skin manifestations, which typically occurs before age 2 years.[26] A study by Amitai and colleagues[9] in 2006 reported that 46% of patients had improvement of the skin lesions within 3 years. Of that 46%, 10% had completely disappeared and the remaining 36% had marked improvement.

Factors that predict which lesions resolve have yet to be identified. However, it is thought that the thickening of the epidermis and dermis associated with natural maturation of the skin plays a role in resolution.[27] Functional maturation of the nervous system at the level of terminal blood vessels within the skin has also been proposed as a mechanism of resolution.[28] This mechanism was reported by Bormann and colleagues[28] in 2001, who, through the use of laser Doppler fluximetry, suggested that CMTC originates from a defect at this level.

Laser therapy has been suggested for the reticulate erythema of CMTC. Sporadic cases have reported improvement, but often the laser type is not indicated. Argon laser therapy has been suggested as a theoretic treatment, but no successful treatments have been reported.[29] Yttrium aluminum garnet laser therapy has been attempted, but without significant success. The large, tortuous, complicated network of distended veins and capillaries of CMTC has been implicated in the lack of response to laser therapy.[27] It has been proposed that treatment with pulsed-dye laser or long pulsed-dye laser could be attempted, but its success has not yet been evaluated.

SUMMARY

CMTC is a rare congenital condition of unknown cause. It is characterized by a pattern of reticulate erythema, known as cutis marmorata, as well as phlebectasia and telangiectasia. Unlike benign cutis marmorata, it does not resolve with warming. CMTC can be associated with several extracutaneous findings, making physical examination a critical component to diagnosis. Subcriteria addressing the occurrence of macrocephaly as a common extracutaneous finding has been a topic of much debate and discussion. Diagnostic criteria have been suggested to assist in the diagnosis of CMTC, but its diagnostic validity has not yet been fully established. Prognosis for patients with CMTC can vary, with routine multidisciplinary follow-up suggested within the first years of life to monitor for any new-onset abnormalities.

REFERENCES

1. Schwartz RA, Zalewska A, Onder M et al. Cutis marmorata telangiectatica congenita. Available at: http://emedicine.medscape.com/article/1086221. Accessed July 7, 2015.
2. Kienast AK, Hoeger PH. Cutis marmorata telangiectatica congenita: a prospective study of 27 cases and review of the literature with proposal of diagnostic criteria. Clin Exp Dermatol 2009;34(3):319–23.

3. De Maio C, Pomero A, Delogu A, et al. Cutis marmorata telangiectatica congenita in a preterm female newborn: case report and review of the literature. Pediatr Med Chir 2014;36(4):161–6.
4. Petrozzi JW, Rahn EK, Mofenson H, et al. Cutis marmorata telangiectatica congenita. Arch Dermatol 1970;101(1):74–7.
5. South DA, Jacobs AH. Cutis marmorata telangiectatica congenita (congenital generalized phlebectasia). J Pediatr 1978;93:944–9.
6. Devillers AC, de Waard-van der Spek FB, Oranje AP. Cutis marmorata telangiectatica congenita: clinical features in 35 cases. Arch Dermatol 1999;135(1):34–8.
7. Kurczynski TW. Hereditary cutis marmorata telangiectatica congenita. Pediatrics 1982;70(1):52–3.
8. Andreev VC, Pramatarov K. Cutis marmorata telangiectatica congenita in two sisters. Br J Dermatol 1979;101:345–50.
9. Amitai DB, Fichman S, Merlob P, et al. Cutis marmorata telangiectatica congenita: clinical findings in 85 patients. Pediatr Dermatol 2000;17(2):100–4.
10. Hinek A, Jain S, Taylor G, et al. High copper levels and increased elastolysis in a patient with cutis marmorata teleangiectasia congenita. Am J Med Genet A 2008; 146A:2520–7.
11. Rogers M, Poyzer KG. Cutis marmorata telangiectatica congenita. Arch Dermatol 1982;118:895–9.
12. Fujita M, Darnstadt GL, Dinulos JG. Cutis marmorata telangiectatica congenita with hemangiomatous histopathologic features. J Am Acad Dermatol 2003;48: 950–4.
13. Martinez-Glez V, Romanelli V, Mori MA, et al. Macrocephaly-capillary malformation: analysis of 13 patients and review of diagnostic criteria. Am J Med Genet A 2010;152A(12):3101–6.
14. Toriello HV, Mulliken JB. Accurately renaming macrocephaly-cutis marmorata telangiectatica congenita (M-CMTC) as macrocephaly-capillary malformation (M-CM). Am J Med Genet A 2007;143A:3009.
15. van Steensel MA. Cutis marmorata telangiectatica congenita. Maastricht University Medical Center, The Netherlands: National Organization for Rare Disorders; 2009. Available at: http://rarediseases.org/rare-diseases/cutis-marmorata-telangiectatica-congenita/. Accessed July 17, 2015.
16. Levy R, Lam JM. Cutis marmorata telangiectatica congenita: a mimicker of a common disorder. CMAJ 2011;183(4):E249–51.
17. Ponnurangam VN, Paramasivam V. Cutis marmorata telangiectatica congenita. Indian Dermatol Online J 2014;5(1):80–2.
18. Pehr K, Moroz B. Cutis marmorata telangiectatica congenita: long-term follow-up, review of the literature, and report of a case in conjunction with congenital hypothyroidism. Pediatr Dermatol 1993;10:6–11.
19. Van Schaik SM, Reneman L, Engelen M, et al. Strokelike episodes and cutis marmorata telangiectatica congenita. J Child Neurol 2015;30(1):129–32.
20. Moore CA, Toriello HV, Abuelo DN, et al. Macrocephaly-cutis marmorata telangiectatica congenita: a distinct disorder with developmental delay and connective tissue abnormalities. Am J Med Genet 1997;70:67–73.
21. Gonzalez ME, Burk CJ, Barbouth CJ, et al. Macrocephaly-capillary malformation: a report of three cases and review of the literature. Pediatr Dermatol 2009;26(3): 342–6.
22. Wright DR, Frieden IJ, Orlow SJ, et al. The misnomer "macrocephaly-cutis marmorata telangiectatica congenital syndrome": report of 12 new cases and

support for revising the name to macrocephaly-capillary malformation. Arch Dermatol 2009;145(3):287–93.

23. Oduber C, van de horst C, Henk Sillevis Smitt J, et al. A proposal for classification of entities combining vascular malformation and deregulated growth. Eur J Med Genet 2011;54:262–71.
24. Dupont C. Cutis marmorata telangiectatica congenita (Van Lohuizen's syndrome). Br J Dermatol 1977;97:437–9.
25. Picasia DD, Esterly NB. Cutis marmorata telangiectatica congenita: report of 22 cases. J Am Acad Dermatol 1989;20:1098–104.
26. Hu IJ, Chen MT, Tai HC, et al. Cutis marmorata telangiectatica congenita with gangrenous ulceration and hypovolaemic shock. Eur J Pediatr 2005;164:411–3.
27. Mazereeuw-Hautier J, Carel-Caneppele S, Bonafe JL. Cutis marmorata telangiectatica congenita: report of two persistent cases. Pediatr Dermatol 2002;19(6): 506–9.
28. Bormann G, Wohlrab J, Fischer M, et al. Cutis marmorata telangiectatica congenita: laser Doppler fluximetry evidence for a functional nervous defect. Pediatr Dermatol 2001;18:110–3.
29. Kennedy C, Oranje AP, Keizer K, et al. Cutis marmorata telangiectatica congenita. Int J Dermatol 1992;31:249–52.

Biopsy and Suture Methodology

Jonathan Soh, BS[a], Christie Riemer, BS[b], Theodore Alkousakis, MD[c],
Ramin Fathi, MD[c],*

KEYWORDS

- Dermatology • Punch biopsy • Shave biopsy • Excisional biopsy • Curettage
- Suture

KEY POINTS

- Skin biopsy is a powerful tool to help practitioners diagnose and treat dermatologic conditions.
- The most common types of biopsies are the shave, punch, curette, and incisional and excisional biopsies.
- Before obtaining any biopsy, it is important to consider the site, morphology, and suspected pathology of a lesion, as well as patient preferences and skin characteristics.

INTRODUCTION

A large number of diagnoses in dermatology are made based on clinicopathologic correlation. Providers routinely develop broad differential diagnoses based on gross findings that are narrowed down after histologic examination and reports from pathologists. Fortunately, providers have access to cutaneous lesions and can biopsy those in question. Properly conducted biopsies may be curative (if negative margins are obtained), and can provide an early diagnosis to better determine course of therapy. Skin biopsies are used in a number of common scenarios outlined in this article (**Box 1**). The most common reasons to biopsy are for inflammatory diseases and malignancy.[1] To maximize tissue sampling and patient satisfaction, familiarity with different types of biopsy techniques is important. Clinicians must also appreciate the indications for each type of biopsy based on different skin lesion appearance and patient characteristics.

The authors have no financial interests or conflicts of interest to disclose.

[a] Department of Dermatology, University of Rochester School of Medicine and Dentistry, Box 427, Rochester, NY 14627, USA; [b] Department of Dermatology, Michigan State University College of Human Medicine, 15 Michigan Street Northeast, Grand Rapids, MI 49503, USA; [c] Department of Dermatology, University of Colorado Denver, 1665 Aurora Court, Anschutz Cancer Pavilion, Aurora, CO 80045, USA
* Corresponding author.
E-mail address: ramin.fathi@ucdenver.edu

Box 1
Common scenarios for skin biopsy

a. Diagnose or rule out a diagnosis that shares similar clinical appearance with another (ie, inflammatory disorders)

b. Histologically confirm a clinical diagnosis that requires treatment (ie, basal cell carcinoma)

c. Surveillance for new disease in special populations (ie, keratinocyte cancers in those who are chronically immunosuppressed)

d. Monitor disease progression or response to treatment

e. Curative excision of a tumor or nonmalignant lesion (ie, tumor removed with histologically negative margins)

f. Diagnose underlying systemic disease suspected from cutaneous findings (ie, genetic syndromes, amyloidosis, connective tissue disorders)

BIOPSY INDICATIONS, CONTRAINDICATIONS, AND GENERAL POINTS TO CONSIDER

Biopsies are a relatively benign procedure that can help provide clinicians with a diagnosis or guidance in decision-making. Overall, indications for biopsy include cases of uncertain diagnosis, or instances when a diagnosis must be determined before definitive treatment is begun. Although there are no absolute contraindications for minor dermatologic procedures, some patient scenarios require special consideration. A thorough examination of the patient's history, comorbidities, and lesion properties will help predict the biopsy's histology interpretation, infection risk, and scar formation. **Table 1** outlines common patient scenarios that may require special consideration.

To best sample underlying skin pathology, the age and evolution of the lesion and location of the biopsy should be considered.[2,3] **Table 2** details the types of biopsies to obtain for common skin morphologies and when in the disease process to sample these lesions.

BIOPSY METHODOLOGY

Seven of the most common biopsy techniques and indications for use in everyday dermatologic practice are outlined in **Table 3**. Each has associated indications and differs in quality and amount of tissue obtained. Regardless of the type of biopsy, systematic steps define any dermatologic procedure.[3] Patient and procedure preparation, anesthesia, biopsy technique and specimen processing, hemostasis, closure, and wound care are reviewed here.

Pre-biopsy Steps

Obtain patient consent. Mark and confirm the site with the patient, and photograph the marked area next to a patient label or identifier (include some surface anatomy in the frame for future reference). Next, fill out pathology requisition forms. These steps are critical for a successful biopsy, subsequent pathology interpretation, and clinical management.[4,5]

Anesthesia

The next step is to anesthetize the area. Local anesthesia is adequate for dermatologic procedures. These drugs consist of a hydrophobic aromatic group and a hydrophilic amine group. Anesthetics are classified into either esters or amides based on which

Table 1
Special considerations for biopsies

Genital areas and mucosa	Heal well due to high vascularity and quick skin turnover
Anatomically significant areas	Be aware of nerves and vessels of the head and neck (ie, temporal and facial nerves, spinal accessory nerve, temporal and thyroid arteries)
History of keloid	More likely in darkly pigmented skin; shoulders, earlobes, upper arm, chest Prophylactic pressure dressings, silicone gel sheets, imiquimod with mixed results[26,27]
History of hypertrophic scar	Common in areas of high skin tension: shoulders, chest, neck, knees ankles Promote rapid reepithelialization (<10–14 d) and wound hygiene, primary closure under little tension[28]
Pregnancy	Lidocaine with and without epinephrine Class B (no risk to humans) No reported cases of harm from electrocautery Defer elective procedures until after delivery If melanoma, careful excision should be considered during pregnancy[29]
Site overlying bone prominences	Tendency for chronic inflammation and epidermal hyperplasia
Sites and populations with higher risk of infection	Below the waist, ulcerated lesions, lip, ear, groin, inpatient samples, patients who smoke, patients with diabetes[25]
Sites on the back, ventral forearms	Scars tend to stretch with time
Suspected infectious component	Send part of sample to microbiology to avoid taking multiple biopsies
Patient currently treating the lesion	Biopsy after 1 wk free from treatment
Alopecia	Obtain 2 punch biopsies: 1 for vertical pathology sections, 1 for horizontal
Warfarin, aspirin, nonsteroidal anti-inflammatory drug use	Severe complications in <2% of cases, no significant difference from control subjects[30]

respective group joins the hydrophobic and hydrophilic groups. Esters consist of procaine, cocaine, and tetracaine. Amide anesthetics (lidocaine, prilocaine, bupivacaine, mepivacaine, and ropivacaine) are the most commonly used agents in dermatologic practice.[6,7] Time of onset, duration of action, and maximum dosages are stated in **Table 4**. Pediatric dosing for lidocaine should be 80% of the maximum dose.[8] If a true allergy-to-amide anesthetic exists, an ester class can be used.

Topical formulations are used to reduce the pain of an injection in pediatric and anxious adult patients; 1% lidocaine is the most commonly used local anesthetic for infiltration. Technique varies slightly based on the type of biopsy performed; however, the goal is to provide anesthesia to all levels of the epidermis, dermis, and subcutis that will be biopsied. General practice principles are stated in **Box 2**.

For most punch and shave biopsies, the amount of local anesthetic required is small (1–3 mL) and can be injected into the dermis. Despite being more painful, intradermal injections have a quicker onset of analgesia than subcutaneous injections. The addition of epinephrine causes vasoconstriction, which aids in hemostasis and analgesia

Table 2
Morphology and chronicity guide where to biopsy within a lesion

Morphology	Timing	Lesion Location
1. Tumor and inflammatory	Early, well-defined lesions	Center
2. Vesiculobullous, pustular	Early, small and intact lesions	• Entire lesion • Perilesional skin if for immunofluorescence
3. Ulcer	Early, small lesion	Leading edge with perilesional skin, avoid necrotic areas
4. Generalized, polymorphic	Active, well-defined lesions	• Center of any representative lesion • Upper extremity preferred over lower extremity
5. Vasculitis	Early lesions	Palpable purpura or center of representative lesion
6. Annular	Active lesions	Raised or leading edge
7. Urticaria	Active lesions within 3 d	Center of representative lesion
8. Alopecia	Active lesions	Hairless, inflamed areas
9. Fungus	Active, untreated lesions	Raised, scaly border

prolongation. Epinephrine requires up to 15 minutes to achieve maximum effects. Therefore, immediate biopsies can be conducted with or without epinephrine.[9]

Biopsy Technique

Biopsy techniques are described as follows. Incisional and excisional biopsy techniques are pictured in **Fig. 1**.[3,10,11]

Curettage

Curettage is the most superficial mode of biopsy; results are generally insufficient for pathology diagnosis, as tissue architecture can easily be destroyed. To perform, the patient is prepped and tray prepared with curette (3–5 mm, various types available: cup-shaped, spoon type, or ring type), gauze, electrocautery, Vaseline, and clean dressing. Caution is required when using a ring-type curette, as it can easily damage thin skin.

Inject 1 to 3 mL lidocaine intradermally to elevate the lesion with a wheal formation. The curette is held in the dominant hand, like a pencil, fingertips near the neck of the cutting edge. The nondominant hand stretches surrounding skin for better traction. With moderate pressure, one smooth, downward scraping motion is used to remove the lesion. Depending on type of curette and appearance of lesion, final biopsy may be an epithelial sheet or ball of tissue. Hemostasis is usually obtained by direct pressure or electrocautery. This type of lesion heals by secondary intention; scarring is usually minimal.

Snip/scissors

This is a quick and efficient method to biopsy pedunculated lesions. Set up includes Iris or Gradle scissors and toothed forceps. Local anesthetic is injected into the upper dermis, elevating the base of the lesion with a wheal formation. If the lesion has a very narrow peduncle, this procedure can be completed without anesthesia.

Pick up the lesion with forceps to provide slight traction (excess pulling can lift the skin base and result in a wider cut into uninvolved tissue). With scissors flush to the skin surface, transect the lesion stalk. Firm pressure should provide sufficient

Table 3
Description and indications of 7 types of biopsies

Biopsy Type	Description of Use	Clinical Indication
1. Curettage	Most superficial sampling method; typically used for removal of lesion, not to obtain a pathology specimen	Epidermal lesions, that is molluscum contagiosum, viral warts, seborrheic keratosis (SK), actinic keratosis (AK), small superficial basal cell carcinoma (BCC), solar keratoses
2. Snip/Scissors	Quick, easy removal of lesions with a stalk	Pedunculated lesions, skin tags
3. Shave	Captures epidermal or papillary dermal lesions, elevated lesions	Viral warts, SK, intradermal/compound nevi, neurofibroma • Exophytic benign growths, AK, superficial neoplasms • SUBOPTIMAL for: deep margin visualization (ie, Bowens vs squamous cell carcinoma) or suspected melanoma or acral areas with thick stratum corneum
4. Saucerization	Similar to shave biopsy, passes through reticular dermis and/or subcutis	Similar to shave biopsy
5. Punch/"Core"	Standard for evaluating inflammatory conditions	Inflammatory dermal or subcutaneous lesions, panniculitis, alopecia, nail biopsies
6. Incisional	Partial sampling of the lesion; depth of subcutaneous layer, preserves lateral margins; used for diagnostic, not therapeutic purposes	Cutaneous tumors, epidermoid cysts, lipomas, Mohs scheduled for future
7. Excision in toto	Therapeutic removal of entire lesion with margins	Suspected invasive melanoma, clinically typical BCC, Mohs for confirmed malignancy, cosmetic benign subepidermal

hemostasis in most cases. Antihemorrhagic solutions (ie, aluminum chloride, ferric sulfate, silver nitrate) and electrodessication can be used if bleeding continues. Most wounds will best heal by secondary intention and leave a small hypopigmented macule.

Shave

This method is frequently used and is excellent for suspected epidermal and papillary dermis pathology; however, shave biopsies are suboptimal for pigmented lesions suspicious for melanoma.

To perform, prep the site and stand with a double-edge or single-edge flexible razor (most commonly used) or #15 blade, and toothed forceps. Inject 1 to 3 mL of local anesthesia intradermally to form a raised wheal, elevating the lesion from surrounding skin. Apply pressure with the nondominant hand to stretch the skin taut. The flexible blade is held between the thumb and index finger of the dominant hand. The blade should be gently bent with a semi-curvilinear shape. Note that the angle of the blade

Table 4
Local anesthesia onset, duration and dosages

Anesthetics	Onset, min	Duration Without Epinephrine, min	Duration with Epinephrine, min	Dosage without Epinephrine, mg/Kg/ Maximum Total Dose, mg	Dosage with Epinephrine, mg/Kg/ Maximum Total Dose, mg
Amides					
Lidocaine	Immediate	30–120	60–400	4/350	7/500
Bupivacaine	5–8	120–140	240–480	2/175	3/225
Prilocaine	5–6	30–120	60–400	6/400	8/600
Mepivacaine	3–20	30–120	30–120	4/300	7/500
Esters					
Procaine	5	15–30	30–90	7/500	9/600

determines the depth of the cut. More concavity equates a deeper cut. Hold the blade parallel to the skin surface at the base of the lesion. Use a smooth sawing, side-to-side motion to cut. Control bleeding with pressure, electrocautery, or chemical hemostasis. Wounds heal by secondary intention.

Saucerization

This method is used to diagnose pathology involving the epidermis and upper dermis. The setup is the same as that for a shave biopsy (flexible single-edge or double-edge razor blade, or #15 blade, toothed forceps). Inject 1 to 3 mL of intradermal local anesthesia to elevate the lesion with a wheal formation.

Again, the nondominant hand stretches the surrounding skin to make the lesion taut. The dominant hand holds the razor blade between the thumb and index or middle finger. The depth of a saucerization is obtained by flexing the blade with steady pressure between the fingers. When the desired concavity of the blade is obtained, a gentle sawing motion is applied at the base of the wheal and is continued until the entire lesion is removed. If using a #15 blade, start perpendicular to the skin surface and reach the intended depth (dermis), then use a smooth sawing motion as you

Box 2
Local anesthesia administration tips to reduce pain and maximize effectiveness

- Infiltrate the tissue slowly using smallest-gauge needle (28 or 30)
- Cool the skin with ice before cleaning with alcohol
- Pinch the skin around the lesion to raise the lesion
- Massaging the lesion can help distribute the anesthetic
- Use anesthetic that is at room temperature
- Inject into subcutis versus dermis to reduce the amount of stretch and subsequent pain
- Subcutaneous injections have slower onset of action than intradermal
- Beware of inadvertent intravascular infiltration and the signs and symptoms of central nervous and cardiovascular system toxicity

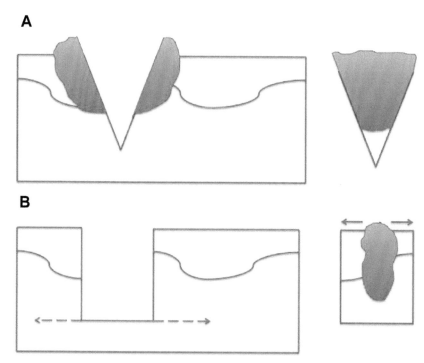

Fig. 1. (*A*) Incisional biopsy: diagnostic sampling of a lesion to any desired depth. Wedge-shaped tissue specimen is obtained and sent to pathology. (*B*) Excisional biopsy: diagnostic and therapeutic removal of a lesion to any desired depth. Note vertical walls of wound, margins from clinical apparent lesion (*solid arrows*) and undermining at the same level as the base of the excision (*broken arrows*).

turn the blade horizontally and continue parallel to the skin surface. Residual edges of the lesion can be curetted off.

Firm pressure should be sufficient to achieve hemostasis in most cases. Antihemorrhagic solutions (ie, aluminum chloride, ferric sulfate, silver nitrate) and electrodessication may be applied if bleeding continues. The wound is typically left to close by secondary intention. Reepithelization occurs over 1 to 2 weeks and will leave a hypopigmented macule or slight depression.

Punch/core

Most commonly used to assess deep dermal pathology, punch biopsies help capture inflammatory processes (ie, alopecia, panniculitis). The diameter of the punch tool cutting edge determines the volume of tissue sampled. The average biopsy size is with a 4-mm punch. If a subcutaneous disease process is suspected (panniculitis), a larger punch should be used. Cosmetically sensitive areas may be sampled with smaller diameters.

To perform, obtain a disposable punch tool, tissue holders, tissue scissors, violet skin marker, and suture material. Prepare the area and outline the desired biopsy site. The site will be closed by primary closure; therefore, map out the direction of the skin tension lines in the area. Sutures will be placed perpendicularly to suture lines.

Inject 1 to 3 mL of local anesthetic superficially and deeper into dermis. To obtain optimal esthetic results, use the nondominant hand to stretch the skin in a perpendicular direction to marked skin tension lines. Push the punch biopsy tool into the lesion using a rotational downward motion. Continue to rotate the tool in one direction with downward pressure until subcutaneous tissue is reached. Avoid back-and-forth twisting motions to maintain epidermal integrity. Remove the tool, and use forceps to gently grab the specimen. Tissue scissors or a razor blade can help remove the lesion at the base to include subcutaneous tissue. Hemostasis and closure are traditionally accomplished with primary closure (4-0 or 5-0 suture, 6-0 for face). Run the sutures perpendicular to skin tension lines and include 1 to 3 interrupted sutures. The final defect will run in parallel with relaxed skin tension lines.

Incisional
This technique may be used to obtain a sampling of the lesion to any desired depth (see **Fig. 1**A). The primary tool is the #15 scalpel blade. With anesthetic, slowly infiltrate the entire dermal compartment that will be removed. Wait up to 15 minutes for maximal onset of the effect of epinephrine.

Start by orienting and marking the long axis of the biopsy site along relaxed skin tension lines. Score the lateral edge of the lesion boundary with a #15 bladed scalpel held perpendicularly to the skin surface. Cut through just the epidermis. The nondominant hand applies traction and skin tightening. Repeat this step on the other nonincised side of the lesion outline.

Retrace the initial scores (one at a time) with firmer, steady pressure to reach the desired depth within the dermis. Gradually angle the blade toward the midline of the lesion so that, when the incisions meet at the base, a wedge-shaped tissue specimen is removed. Apply traction up and away from the skin surface with forceps and trim any remaining adhesions to free the lesion from the surrounding tissue.

Hemostasis is achieved with focal electrodessication of the wound bed. Large arteries may require a figure-of-eight tie off. Close the wound with interrupted deep dermal or subcuticular stitches (absorbable, 4-0 or 5-0 suture). The overlying epidermis is closed with interrupted nylon or polypropylene monofilament (6-0 for face, 4-0 and 5-0 for other sites). The patient should be left with a thin hypopigmented linear scar; however, inform the patient that spreading of the scar can occur over areas of high skin tension, such as the back and trunk.

Excisional (in toto)
This method provides therapeutic and diagnostic removal of an entire lesion. Often, it may be used to remove perilesional skin for margin analysis (see **Fig. 1**B). The primary tool is the #15 scalpel blade. Infiltrate local anesthetic beyond the entire dermal compartment to be removed, as tissue undermining will be required before closure. Over 10 to 15 minutes, slowly inject anesthetic agent to allow full pain control and vasoconstrictive properties.

Start by orienting the long axis of the cut along relaxed skin tension lines, and outline a fusiform incision shape. Score the lateral edge of the lesion boundary with a #15 scalpel blade held perpendicularly to the skin surface. Cut through the epidermis, using the nondominant hand to apply traction. Repeat this step on the other side.

Retrace the initial scores (one at a time) with firmer, steady pressure to reach the desired depth. Unlike the beveled incisions of the incisional biopsy, excisional incisions are made perpendicular to the skin surface all the way to the subcutis or fascia. The 2 sides of the incisions should converge at both apices of the ellipse, and reach the same depth as that in the middle. Apply traction up and away from the skin surface with forceps. The base of the specimen can be dissected away with scissors or a blade, leaving an elliptical excision with uniformly deep vertical walls and a flat base of subcutis or fascia.

Depending on the diagnosis, margins of various sizes must be taken with the lesion[12–14]:

- Well-circumscribed basal cell carcinoma or squamous cell carcinoma (SCC): 3 to 5 mm
- Atypical nevi: 2 to 4 mm
- Melanoma in situ: 5 mm-10 mm
- Invasive melanoma: 10 to 20 mm depending on the depth of invasion

Hemostasis is achieved with focal electrodessication; large arteries may require figure-of-eight tie off. To aid in tension-free closure, undermine the surrounding wound edges with scissors (blunt and sharp dissection) or scalpel. Undermining should be at the same level as the wound base. This process creates a movable unit of skin that will ultimately fill in the resulting defect. Next, close with 1 or 2 layers of interrupted deep dermal or subcuticular sutures (absorbable, 4-0 or 5-0). The overlying epidermis is closed with simple interrupted or continuous nylon or polypropylene monofilament (6-0 for face, 4-0 and 5-0 for other sites). The final wound edges should be opposed and everted slightly to create a flat, thin scar.

Specimen Processing

Once the tissue sample is obtained, it must be sent to pathology in the correct preservative media. Unless an exception is listed (**Table 5**), tissue samples should be immediately fixed in 10% neutral buffered formalin. Confirm that the skin is floating in the solution and is not stuck to the container or cap, where it may desiccate and compromise histologic quality. The tissue specimen and container should be accompanied by the pathology requisition form. The container and form should identically describe correct anatomic location, procedure type, brief clinical history and patient identifiers. There are a number of instances in which very subtle to no pathologic changes are visible on routine hematoxylin-eosin processing.[15] Many skin disease processes also follow identical histologic patterns, and are not discernable without clinical correlation. Therefore, clinical information is critical for the pathologist to render accurate interpretation or guide immunohistochemical stain selection.[2]

Hemostasis

Initial hemostasis should be attempted with sponges and gauze. For smaller biopsies (ie, punch), gauze pressure or primary closure with suture typically provides adequate mechanical hemostasis. Larger procedures, such as incisional biopsies and excisions in toto, should be followed by localized electrocoagulation with the goal of no active bleeding in the wound bed. If a larger vessel is visibly bleeding, the source may be tied off with a figure-of-eight stitch.[16]

Table 5
Tissue specimens and fixation media

Histologic Examination	Fixation Media	Clinical Examples
Hematoxylin-eosin	10% neutral buffered formalin	Most routine biopsies
Direct immunofluorescence	Michel media or saline	Vesiculobullous disease
Flow cytometry	Saline soaked gauze	Lymphoma
Infectious	Viral transport media, bacterial, fungal cultures	Tinea, herpes

Closure

Routine biopsies heal by primary or secondary intention. Primary intention refers to the use of suture material to approximate wound edges. Secondary intention involves leaving the wound open to allow natural granulation and closure. Both types of closure are based on principles of wound healing, granulation tissue formation, and wound contraction. Strengths and indications of each are outlined in **Table 6**. When deciding between primary and secondary closure, wound size and location, patient preference, lifestyle restriction, accessibility for follow-up suture removal, and expectations for scar appearance are taken into account.[17]

A full-thickness stitch or a layered closure may be used for primary closure. A deep dermal suture is placed to approximate subcutaneous fat and dermal tissue, ultimately everting the superficial wound edges ("puckered edge") to create a flat, smooth healed defect as the scar matures. This deep subcutaneous suture is helpful in providing mechanical hemostasis as well. Synthetic absorbable sutures (ie, braided polyglactin or monofilament polydioxanone) remain intact for 8 to 12 weeks, which is the amount of time generally needed for tensile strength to develop. On top of deep dermal sutures, a layer of epidermal nonabsorbable sutures (ie, monofilament nylon or polypropylene) approximate and complete the everted wound edges. Nonabsorbable sutures should be removed to prevent a foreign body reaction, such as granuloma formation. If a biopsy is performed on the face, sutures can be removed after approximately 7 days. Sutures elsewhere on the body can be removed after 2 weeks.

Wound Care

Visible marks, color, and texture tend to improve as scar tissue matures. Vigilant wound care promotes a noncontaminated, debris and desiccation-free healing site. Simple wounds can be treated with mild soap, then dressed with petrolatum and a bandage until sutures are removed or epithelialization has occurred. Debris and crusting should be removed on a regular basis. Keeping the wound moist helps promote reepithelialization and cosmetic appearance.[18]

Table 6
Primary and secondary intention

Type	Description	Indications	Notes
Primary	Approximated wound edges close defect; that is, grafts, side-to-side closures, flaps	• Larger wounds, >8 mm • Punch biopsies	• More fibroblast activity and collagen deposition promote greater tensile strength • Faster healing time • Better patient satisfaction, less pain, fewer dressing changes if >8 mm (no difference <4 mm)
Secondary	Wound is allowed to heal without being closed	• Long commute to appointments • Unavoidable activity, no restrictions	• No suture removal appointment, no activity restrictions • Potential cost saving • Longer healing time

Complications of Biopsy

Despite the relative safety of biopsy, complications can occur.[19] The following sections describe some of these complications.

Hypersensitivity to local anesthetic

True allergic reactions (allergic contact dermatitis, urticaria, anaphylaxis) to local anesthetic or preservative (sulfites and parabens) are rare and reported at less than 1%.[20–22] Most adverse effects (paresthesia, anxiety, tachycardia, dizziness) are pseudoallergic and occur secondary to vasovagal, sympathetic stimulation or systemic toxicity.[23] Although small amounts of local anesthetic are typically used, accidental intravascular injection can lead to central nervous system and cardiovascular toxicity (tachycardia, hypertension, arrhythmia).[6]

Pain to local anesthetics

The sensation of pain arises from the initial stick of the needle, rapid stretch and expansion of the skin (wheal formation), or from the drug itself. To minimize pain, one may attempt to precool the biopsy area with ice before sterilization with an alcohol solution. To decrease pain from wheal formation, withdraw the needle slightly as lidocaine is injected and use only the amount of anesthetic needed to avoid overexpansion of the site. Palmoplantar sites are extremely sensitive; therefore, attempt to inject lidocaine in small amounts before advancing and injecting more. Injecting from dorsal aspect of the extremity is also a possibility if the lesion is located on the sides of the palms or soles. Anesthetic drugs have an acidic pH; although this prolongs shelf life, acidity also stimulates pain. Buffering the anesthetic with sodium bicarbonate can be beneficial.

Bleeding

Certain areas are more prone to bleed (scalp, genital area, atrophic skin). It is important to be aware of large underlying vessels in proximity to the biopsy area. In most cases, bleeding originates from small venules and will respond to 5 minutes of steady pressure. Hemostatic measures can be applied if there is uncontrolled bleeding.

Scarring

Before performing a biopsy, ask about patient history of keloid or hypertrophic scarring. Two vascular plexi exist, one at the border of the papillary and reticular dermis, the other between the reticular dermis and subcutis. There are few vertically oriented vessels that connect the 2 plexi. Biopsies ending at the mid-reticular layer are therefore more susceptible to ischemia, infection, and scarring. It is best to biopsy through the subcutaneous tissue.

Infection

Biopsies and excisions are safe outpatient procedures with low rates of infection of approximately 2%.[24] The size and location (ie, the ear, below waist) of the excision, as well as the patient's smoking history and inpatient versus outpatient status, are considered important factors for infection risk.[25]

SUMMARY

Skin biopsy is a powerful tool to help practitioners diagnose and treat dermatologic conditions. The most common types of biopsies are the shave, punch, curette, and incisional and excisional biopsies. Before obtaining any biopsy, it is important to consider the site, morphology, and suspected pathology of a lesion, as well as patient preferences and skin characteristics. Selecting the appropriate biopsy technique results in better histologic specimens for pathology, better diagnostic capabilities, fewer complications, and greater patient safety and satisfaction. Whether closed by primary or secondary intention, good wound care, patient education, and an awareness of potential complications help round out a smooth biopsy procedure.

REFERENCES

1. Alguire PC, Mathes BM. Skin biopsy techniques for the internist. J Gen Intern Med 1998;13(1):46–54.
2. Sina B, Kao GF, Deng AC, et al. Skin biopsy for inflammatory and common neoplastic skin diseases: optimum time, best location and preferred techniques. A critical review. J Cutan Pathol 2009;36(5):505–10.
3. Sleiman R, Kurban M, Abbas O. Maximizing diagnostic outcomes of skin biopsy specimens. Int J Dermatol 2013;52(1):72–8.
4. Fleischman M, Garcia C. Informed consent in dermatologic surgery. Dermatol Surg 2003;29(9):952–5 [discussion: 955].
5. McGinness JL, Goldstein G. The value of preoperative biopsy-site photography for identifying cutaneous lesions. Dermatol Surg 2010;36(2):194–7.
6. Walsh A, Walsh S. Local anaesthesia and the dermatologist. Clin Exp Dermatol 2011;36(4):337–43.
7. Hruza G. Anesthesia. In: Bolognia J, Jorizzo JL, Schaffer JV, editors. Dermatology. Philadelphia: Elsevier Saunders; 2012. p. 2343–52.
8. McCreight A, Stephan M. Textbook of pediatric emergency procedures. In: King C, Henretig FM, editors. Local and regional anesthesia. 2nd edition. Philadelphia: Lippincott, Williams, & Wilkins; 2008. p. 439–68.
9. Liu S, Carpenter RL, Chiu AA, et al. Epinephrine prolongs duration of subcutaneous infiltration of local anesthesia in a dose-related manner. Correlation with magnitude of vasoconstriction. Reg Anesth 1995;20(5):378–84.
10. Olbricht S. Biopsy techniques and basic excisions. In: Bolognia J, Jorizzo JL, Schaffer JV, editors. Dermatology. Philadelphia: Elsevier Saunders; 2012. p. 2381–97.
11. Affleck A, Colver G. Skin biopsy techniques. In: Robinson JK, editor. Surgery of the skin procedural dermatology. Edinburgh (Scotland); New York: Mosby Elsevier; 2010. p. 165–76, online resource (xvii, 850 p.).
12. Bichakjian CK, Halpern AC, Johnson TM, et al. Guidelines of care for the management of primary cutaneous melanoma. American Academy of Dermatology. J Am Acad Dermatol 2011;65(5):1032–47.
13. Reddy KK, Farber MJ, Bhawan J, et al. Atypical (dysplastic) nevi: outcomes of surgical excision and association with melanoma. JAMA Dermatol 2013;149(8):928–34.
14. Thomas DJ, King AR, Peat BG. Excision margins for nonmelanotic skin cancer. Plast Reconstr Surg 2003;112(1):57–63.
15. Mehregan DR, Dooley VN. How to get the most out of your skin biopsies. Int J Dermatol 2007;46(7):727–33.
16. Palm MD, Altman JS. Topical hemostatic agents: a review. Dermatol Surg 2008;34(4):431–45.
17. Christenson LJ, Phillips PK, Weaver AL, et al. Primary closure vs second-intention treatment of skin punch biopsy sites: a randomized trial. Arch Dermatol 2005;141(9):1093–9.
18. Liu A, Moy RL, Ozog DM. Current methods employed in the prevention and minimization of surgical scars. Dermatol Surg 2011;37(12):1740–6.

19. Nischal U, Nischal K, Khopkar U. Techniques of skin biopsy and practical considerations. J Cutan Aesthet Surg 2008;1(2):107–11.
20. Fisher MM, Pennington JC. Allergy to local anaesthesia. Br J Anaesth 1982;54(8): 893–4.
21. Gall H, Kaufmann R, Kalveram CM. Adverse reactions to local anesthetics: analysis of 197 cases. J Allergy Clin Immunol 1996;97(4):933–7.
22. Batinac T, Sotošek Tokmadžić V, Peharda V, et al. Adverse reactions and alleged allergy to local anesthetics: analysis of 331 patients. J Dermatol 2013;40(7): 522–7.
23. Fiset L, Milgrom P, Weinstein P, et al. Psychophysiological responses to dental injections. J Am Dent Assoc 1985;111(4):578–83.
24. Futoryan T, Grande D. Postoperative wound infection rates in dermatologic surgery. Dermatol Surg 1995;21(6):509–14.
25. Wahie S, Lawrence CM. Wound complications following diagnostic skin biopsies in dermatology inpatients. Arch Dermatol 2007;143(10):1267–71.
26. Berman B, Harrison-Balestra C, Perez OA, et al. Treatment of keloid scars post-shave excision with imiquimod 5% cream: a prospective, double-blind, placebo-controlled pilot study. J Drugs Dermatol 2009;8(5):455–8.
27. Gold MH, Foster TD, Adair MA, et al. Prevention of hypertrophic scars and keloids by the prophylactic use of topical silicone gel sheets following a surgical procedure in an office setting. Dermatol Surg 2001;27(7):641–4.
28. Slemp AE, Kirschner RE. Keloids and scars: a review of keloids and scars, their pathogenesis, risk factors, and management. Curr Opin Pediatr 2006;18(4): 396–402.
29. Richards KA, Stasko T. Dermatologic surgery and the pregnant patient. Dermatol Surg 2002;28(3):248–56.
30. Otley CC, Fewkes JL, Frank W, et al. Complications of cutaneous surgery in patients who are taking warfarin, aspirin, or nonsteroidal anti-inflammatory drugs. Arch Dermatol 1996;132(2):161–6.

Topical Therapy Primer for Nondermatologists

Jolene R. Jewell, MD, Sarah A. Myers, MD*

KEYWORDS

- Topical therapies • Corticosteroids • Antimicrobials • Retinoids
- Nondermatologist providers

KEY POINTS

- Many dermatologic conditions are effectively managed with topical therapies, including topical steroids, antimicrobials, retinoids, keratolytics, and antineoplastics.
- The proper active ingredient, potency, vehicle, quantity of medication, and patient instructions are critical when prescribing topical therapies.
- If a topical therapy is ineffective, clinicians should consider whether the medication is being used properly, whether the diagnosis is correct, and whether the topical may be contributing to the problem.

INTRODUCTION

Topical therapy is critical in the care of patients with cutaneous disease. This article offers a concise catalog of commonly used topical therapies and the included tables and cited publications serve as a toolkit for quick reference. Clinical vignettes are provided to reinforce the basic tenets of topical therapy and highlight basic guidelines for primary care providers.

PART I: TOPICAL MEDICATIONS
Topical Steroids

Regarded as the crux of dermatologic therapy, topical corticosteroids (TCS) are prescribed in up to 21% of dermatology office visits for atopic dermatitis, contact dermatitis, hand dermatitis, and many other cutaneous inflammatory conditions.[1] The proper use of TCS requires consideration of steroid potency, vehicle, and quantity of

This article originally appeared in Medical Clinics of North America, Volume 99, Issue 6, November 2015

Disclosures: The authors have no commercial or financial conflicts of interest or funding sources to disclose.

Department of Dermatology, Duke University Medical Center, DUMC 3852, Durham, NC 27710, USA

* Corresponding author.

E-mail address: sarah.myers@duke.edu

medication. Despite standard Stoughton Vasoconstriction Assay–based potency classification, dermatologists often categorize prescription steroids as high, mid, or low potency.[2] TCS are pregnancy category C, thus low-potency steroids are reserved for severe dermatoses during pregnancy. **Table 1** highlights the topical steroids commonly prescribed by dermatologists.

TCS are generally well tolerated; however, side effect frequency and severity increase with prolonged use and steroid potency. Epidermal atrophy, folliculitis or steroid acne, perioral dermatitis, delayed wound healing, steroid rebound, tachyphylaxis, glaucoma, cataracts, and contact dermatitis are all reversible TCS side effects.[3] Striae development is irreversible, thus the risk of this specific adverse event should always be discussed with patients. Systemic side effects, such as hypothalamic-pituitary-adrenal axis suppression, iatrogenic Cushing syndrome, and growth retardation in children, can occur if TCS are used improperly.

Topical Antimicrobials

Acne, rosacea, periorificial dermatitis, tinea, candidal intertrigo, and scabies are frequently treated with topical antimicrobials. Most of the medications discussed here are available in generic formulations and some are available over the counter (OTC), as indicated in **Table 2**. When recommending an OTC medication, instruct patients to check ingredient lists because some brands manufacture similarly named products with different active ingredients.

Topical antimicrobials are often used for basic wound care; however, dermatologists generally recommend petrolatum use to maintain a moist wound-healing environment. A frequently cited randomized controlled trial from 1996 showed the absence of a statistically significant difference in infection rate when petrolatum versus bacitracin was used postoperatively. Further, petrolatum is cheaper than commercially available antibacterial ointments.[4] If an antibacterial ointment is indicated for a superficial skin infection, mupirocin is preferred because of lower risk of allergic contact dermatitis.

Topical Acne, Rosacea, and Psoriasis Medications

Mild to moderate comedonal and inflammatory acne can be effectively treated with topical medications. Many of the topicals listed in **Table 3** are used in conjunction with antimicrobials to improve efficacy and patient adherence. It should be emphasized that these treatments prevent new lesions from forming and thus need to be used on a regular basis for 6 to 8 weeks before efficacy can be assessed. Similarly, acne medications control acne and patients should be warned that their acne may flare if topicals are discontinued. Oral antibiotics and isotretinoin are typically reserved for severe nodulocystic acne with scarring or chest and back involvement. Treating pregnancy-related acne can be challenging because there are few pregnancy category B therapeutics, with the exception of azelaic acid, topical clindamycin, and topical erythromycin. Pregnant patients should be informed that OTC benzoyl peroxide and salicylic acid face washes are technically pregnancy category C.

It can be difficult to distinguish acne from rosacea in some patients. Dermatologists rely on the presence of comedones to suggest the diagnosis of acne rather than rosacea, and patients with rosacea tend to have more sensitive skin. Erythematotelangiectatic rosacea responds best to pulsed dye laser but some patients report significant improvement in flushing with topical brimonidine gel use.[8] Papulopustular rosacea responds well to topical metronidazole, azelaic acid, and newly available topical ivermectin. Ocular rosacea and severe inflammatory rosacea require oral antibiotic use. Phymatous rosacea responds poorly to topicals and often requires cosmetic surgery or laser treatment.[9]

Psoriatic plaques can be treated with topical steroids, but steroid-sparing agents have a special role in refractory disease and intertriginous sites. Unlike topical steroids, the topical calcineurin inhibitors (TCIs), tacrolimus and pimecrolimus, can be applied chronically for psoriasis or atopic dermatitis on the face, axillae, and inguinal folds without causing atrophy. Calcipotriene, a vitamin D analogue, is a similarly safe and effective alternative psoriasis therapeutic. Topical retinoids are traditionally reserved for acne treatment but tazarotene, specifically, is useful for thinning psoriatic plaques. Steroid-sparing medications can be expensive, thus generics should be prescribed when possible. If a generic medication is unavailable, often manufacturer coupons can be found online or via GoodRx.

Topicals for Actinic Keratoses and Nonmelanoma Skin Cancers

Treatment of actinic keratoses (AKs) is indicated because of the risk of progression to squamous cell carcinoma. Cryotherapy is most commonly used but field therapy with a topical can be helpful if a patient has numerous lesions in a localized area. 5-Fluorouracil is the most commonly used topical but all 4 medications in **Table 4** have similar reported efficacies for AK clearance if used properly.[10,11] Dermatologist recommendations on treatment frequency and duration vary but all patients should be warned regarding expected redness and irritation of the treated site. It can be helpful to show patients representative photographs of what they are likely to experience with adequate treatment. Exuberant reactions are common and can be managed by holding treatment for several days and starting a low-potency topical steroid. If field therapy for AKs is recommended, patients should follow up to ensure resolution of concerning lesions. If treatment of nonmelanoma skin cancers with topicals is being considered, a dermatology referral should be entertained.

PART II: CASES
Case 1

A 36-year-old man presents to clinic in February with an extremely pruritic rash on the upper back, arms, and lower legs, as shown in **Fig. 1**. He has been using topical diphenhydramine, which seemed to worsen his symptoms. You astutely diagnose the patient with asteatotic eczema and prescribe a 15-g tube of triamcinolone 0.1% cream for the patient to use twice daily. The patient leaves the clinic with his prescription but promptly calls your clinic the next day stating that the medication burns and he has already used the entire tube. What went wrong?

- Vehicle selection is a critical component of prescribing TCS and can greatly affect patient adherence, as shown in this case. Cream vehicles contain preservatives that can burn when applied to skin with impaired barrier function. The patient would have less burning if an ointment had been prescribed.
- An adequate amount of medication must be prescribed to treat the patient. As a general rule, it takes 30 g to coat an average-sized person from head to toe once. This patient would require 10 to 15 g per application to treat his rash on the back, arms, and legs. Topical steroids are used twice daily, thus he would need 30 g of triamcinolone per day. Commonly used topical steroids such as triamcinolone can be prescribed in 454-g (1 pound) jars.
- Topical diphenhydramine should have been discontinued. OTC topical antipruritics and analgesics can cause allergic and irritant contact dermatitis, which contribute to the patient's itching and burning.

Table 1
Topical corticosteroids commonly used by dermatologists

Potency	Generic Name	Concentration (%)	Vehicles	Brand Names (Vehicles)	Notes
High (class I/II)	Clobetasol propionate	0.05	Cream Foam Gel Lotion Ointment Shampoo Solution Spray	Clobex (lotion, shampoo, spray) Cormax (ointment, solution) Olux (foam) Temovate (cream, gel, ointment, solution)	Most potent topical steroid. Reserved for psoriasis, lichen sclerosus, discoid lupus, and other severe dermatoses. Foam, shampoo, and solution vehicles are useful for scalp psoriasis
	Halobetasol	0.05	Cream Ointment	Ultravate (cream, ointment)	—
	Betamethasone dipropionate	0.05	Cream Lotion Ointment	—	Available in combination products with calcipotriene or clotrimazole
	Fluocinonide	0.05 0.1	Cream Gel Ointment Solution	Lidex Vanos (cream)	Often referred to by brand name Lidex. Solution vehicle useful for scalp psoriasis. The 0.1% concentration only available in cream vehicle
Medium (class III/IV)	Triamcinolone	0.025 0.1 0.5	Cream Ointment Lotion	Trianex (0.05% ointment)	Most commonly used in 0.1% concentration. Lotion only available in 0.025% and 0.1%. Available in combination product with nystatin
	Betamethasone valerate	0.1	Cream Lotion Ointment Foam	Luxiq (0.12% foam)	Foam vehicle useful for scalp psoriasis. Do not confuse with betamethasone dipropionate, which is high potency
	Desoximetasone	0.05 0.25	Cream Gel Ointment Spray	Topicort	Preferred topical corticosteroid for patients with allergic contact dermatitis. Spray available in 0.25% and gel available in 0.05%

Potency	Drug	Concentration (%)	Brand (formulations)	Formulations	Notes
Low (class V/VI)	Fluocinolone	0.025 0.01	Capex (shampoo) Derma-Smoothe/FS (body oil, scalp oil) Synalar (cream, ointment, solution)	Body oil Cream Ointment Scalp oil Shampoo Solution	Oil vehicle useful for scalp psoriasis in patients with dry, coarse hair. Do not confuse with fluocinonide, which is high potency. 0.025% only available in cream and ointment
	Hydrocortisone valerate	0.2	Westcort	Cream Ointment	Note that hydrocortisone valerate at 0.2% is higher potency than hydrocortisone 1%
	Desonide	0.05	Desonate (gel) Desowen (cream, lotion, ointment) Verdeso (foam)	Cream Foam Gel Lotion Ointment	Often used in combination with ketoconazole 2% cream for seborrheic dermatitis
Least (class VII)	Hydrocortisone	0.5 1 2.5	Hytone (1, 2.5% cream) Texacort (2.5% solution)	Cream Lotion Ointment Solution	Lowest potency topical steroid. Available at 1% concentration in many OTC products, such as Cortizone-10 and Cortaid. The 2.5% concentration requires prescription

Abbreviation: OTC, over the counter.

Table 2
Topical antimicrobials commonly used by dermatologists

Antimicrobial Class	Generic Name	Concentration (%)	Vehicles	Brand Names (Vehicles)	Notes
Antibacterial	BPO	2.5–10	Cream Gel Pledget Wash	Numerous OTC preparations available, including PanOxyl, Clean and Clear, and AcneFree	Available in combination products with adapalene, clindamycin, and erythromycin. Bleaches towels/clothing if not rinsed thoroughly
	Clindamycin	1	Foam Gel Lotion Solution	Cleocin T (gel, lotion, solution) Clindagel (gel) Evoclin (foam)	Available in combination products with BPO and tretinoin. Use with BPO wash to prevent bacterial resistance[5]
	Dapsone	5	Gel	Aczone	Newer acne topical. There has been a case report of methemoglobinemia with topical dapsone use[6]
	Metronidazole	0.75 1	Cream Gel Lotion	MetroCream (cream) MetroGel (1% gel) MetroLotion (lotion) Noritate (cream)	Most commonly used for rosacea and periorificial dermatitis
	Mupirocin	2	Cream Ointment	Bactroban Centany (ointment)	Used TID and for MRSA decolonization. Preferred to because of decreased risk of allergic contact dermatitis
	Sulfacetamide-sulfur	10; 2–5	Cream Foam Lotion Suspension Wash	Klaron (10% lotion) Rosanil (10%/5% wash)	Used for acne, rosacea, and seborrheic dermatitis

Category	Generic name	%	Formulation	Brand (formulation)	Notes
Antifungal	Clotrimazole	1	Cream Solution	Lotrimin AF (cream) Fungicure (solution)	OTC. First-line use for candidal intertrigo because it also has some coverage for dermatophytes
	Econazole	1	Cream Foam	Ecoza (foam)	Can be more expensive than OTC antifungals depending on insurance
	Efinaconazole	10	Solution	Jublia	New topical therapy for onychomycosis, used daily for 48 wk
	Ketoconazole	1 2	Cream Gel Foam Shampoo	Extina (foam) Nizoral AD (1% shampoo) Nizoral (shampoo) Xolegel (gel)	Ketoconazole 1% shampoo is OTC, 2% requires a prescription
	Terbinafine	1	Cream Gel Spray	Lamisil AT (cream, gel, spray)	Fungicidal. First-line OTC topical for tinea pedis
Antiparasitic	Ivermectin	1	Cream	Soolantra	Increasingly being used for rosacea by dermatologists[7]
	Permethrin	1 5	Lotion Cream	Elimite (5% cream) Nix (1% lotion is OTC)	For scabies, recommend 5% cream from neck to toes overnight with repeat application in 14 d

Abbreviations: BPO, benzoyl peroxide; MRSA, methicillin-resistant *Staphylococcus aureus*; TID, 3 times a day.

Table 3
Topicals commonly used by dermatologists for acne, rosacea, and psoriasis

Dermatosis	Generic Name	Concentration (%)	Vehicles	Brand Names (Vehicles)	Notes
Acne	Tretinoin	0.025 0.05 0.1	Cream Gel Solution	There are numerous brand name products with varying concentrations and vehicles, the most commonly referred to is Retin-A. Recommend prescribing the generic	Advise patients to evenly apply a pea-sized amount to the entire face, 10–15 min after washing. May cause redness and scaling. Start 2–3 times per week and increase to nightly as tolerated
	Adapalene	0.1 0.3 (gel)	Cream Gel Lotion	Differin	Regarded as potentially less irritating than tretinoin, would use for patients with sensitive skin
	Tazarotene	0.05 0.1	Cream Gel Foam	Avage (0.1% cream) Fabior (0.1% foam) Tazorac (cream, gel)	Can be used for psoriasis as well
	Azelaic acid	15 20	Gel	Azelex (20%) Finacea (15%)	Pregnancy category B. Can be expensive because generic unavailable. Also used for rosacea
	Salicylic acid	2–3	Wash Shampoo	Numerous OTC washes available, including Neutrogena, Aveeno, and Clean and Clear	Can be used for warts at higher concentrations (17%–40%)
Rosacea	Brimonidine	0.33	Gel	Mirvaso	An alpha-2 agonist used qAM to decrease flushing associated with rosacea via vasoconstriction
Psoriasis	Calcipotriene	0.005	Cream Foam Ointment Solution	Calcitrene (ointment) Dovonex (cream, solution) Sorilux (foam)	Works well in combination with topical steroids for psoriasis vulgaris or as monotherapy for inverse psoriasis
	Tacrolimus	0.03 0.1	Ointment	Protopic	TCI commonly used for dermatitis or psoriasis on the face or intertriginous areas
	Pimecrolimus	1	Cream	Elidel	TCI commonly used for dermatitis or psoriasis on the face or intertriginous areas
	Ammonium lactate	12	Cream Lotion	Lac-Hydrin AmLactin (OTC)	Keratolytic. Used on scaly plaques. Also helpful for retention hyperkeratosis in elderly patients
	Urea	35 40 50	Cream Foam Gel Ointment Solution	Gordon's Urea (40% ointment)	Lower concentration creams are available OTC. Can be used for warts and nail removal as well. Irritating if used on normal skin

Abbreviations: qAM, every morning; TCI, topical calcineurin inhibitor.

Table 4
Topicals commonly used by dermatologists for AKs and nonmelanoma skin cancers

Generic Name	Concentration (%)	Brand Names	FDA Approved Use	Off-label Use	Notes
5-FU	0.5 1 2 5	Carac (0.5% cream) Efudex (2% solution, 5% cream) Fluoroplex (1% cream)	AKs • BID ×2–4 wk Superficial BCC • BID ×3–6 wk	SCC in situ • BID × 12 wk	Do not confuse with the topical steroid fluocinonide. Only 5% is FDA approved for treatment of superficial BCC
Diclofenac	3	Solaraze (gel)	AKs • BID ×60–90 d	—	There are 1%–2% diclofenac gels and solutions used for osteoarthritis
Imiquimod	2.5 3.75 5	Aldara Zyclara (2.5%, 3.75%)	AKs • BIW ×16 wk Superficial BCC • M-F qHS × 16 wk	—	Can also be used for genital warts. Requires longer treatment period than 5-FU
Ingenol mebutate	0.015 0.05	Picato (gel)	AK of face and scalp • 0.015% ×3 d Trunk and Ext • 0.05% ×2 d	—	The shortest treatment period of the topical antineoplastics

Abbreviations: BID, twice a day; BIW, twice a week; Ext, extremities; FDA, US Food and Drug Administration; FU, fluorouracil; M-F, Monday through Friday; qHS, every night at bedtime; SCC, squamous cell carcinoma.

Case 2

An 11-year-old girl with atopic dermatitis presents to clinic with worsening pruritus and rash on the popliteal fossae, as shown in **Fig. 2**. She is currently taking short, lukewarm showers once per day and applying fluocinonide 0.05% ointment twice daily. What other recommendations are appropriate at this time?

- Flares of atopic dermatitis can result from bacterial impetiginization or poor daily skin care. Bacterial impetiginization, if mild, can be treated with dilute bleach baths. Ask the patient to soak for 10 to 15 minutes in a warm tub full of water with one-quarter to one-half a cup of bleach 2 to 3 times per week. The patient may then shower to remove the bleach. If impetiginization is severe, bacterial culture and oral antibiotics may be indicated.
- Daily skin care for patients with atopic dermatitis should be emphasized at every appointment. Recommend daily, short, lukewarm showers with fragrance-free soaps. Immediately after bathing the patient should generously apply an emollient such as a fragrance-free cream, lotion, or petrolatum such as CeraVe,

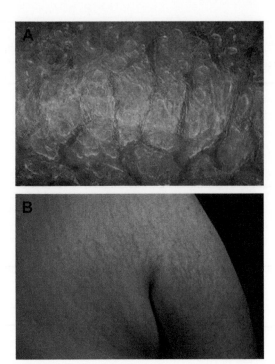

Fig. 1. Asteatotic eczema (eczema craquele). (*A*) The distal lower extremity has obvious inflammation and xerosis with adherent white scales (pseudoichthyosis) as well as crisscross pattern of superficial cracks and fissures said to resemble a dried riverbed. (*B*) When widespread, there can be involvement of the trunk and proximal extremities. Along with the distal lower extremity, the posterior axillary line is a common site for asteatotic eczema. (*From* Reider N, Fritsch O. Other eczematous eruptions. In: Bolognia J, Jorizzo JL, Schaffer JV, editors. Dermatology. Philadelphia: Elsevier Saunders; 2012; with permission.)

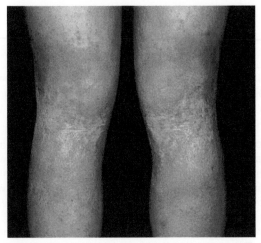

Fig. 2. Flexural involvement in childhood atopic dermatitis. (*From* James WD, Berger TG, Elston DM. Andrews' diseases of the skin: clinical dermatology. Philadelphia: Saunders; 2016; with permission.)

Cetaphil, Aquaphor, or Vaseline. Emollients should be repeated throughout the day as needed in combination with prescribed TCS. As flares resolve, the potency and frequency of TCS use should be decreased, especially in the body folds, because intertriginous skin is at particularly high risk for atrophy.

Case 3

A 42-year-old woman with chronic hand dermatitis presents to clinic with a flare of her eczema, as seen in **Fig. 3**. She has been using betamethasone valerate 0.1% cream twice daily every day for the past month. She reports that the topical steroid used to work but seems to have been less effective for the past week. What other treatment options could be considered?

- If betamethasone valerate 0.1% cream is ineffective, topical steroid potency could be increased to betamethasone dipropionate or clobetasol. The topical steroid vehicle could also be switched from cream to an ointment. More hydrophobic vehicles increase potency via occlusion and enhanced percutaneous absorption (ie, triamcinolone 0.1% ointment is more potent than triamcinolone 0.1% cream).
- When previously steroid-responsive dermatitis flares, clinicians should consider that the topical steroids themselves may be causing contact dermatitis. Recent patch testing results from the North American Contact Dermatitis Group indicates that the incidence of allergic contact dermatitis to TCS is nearly 3.9%.[12] In this situation, the patient could be switched to desoximetasone, an alternative, midpotency topical steroid that does not contain the common allergen propylene glycol.
- Tachyphylaxis should also be considered and the patient may benefit from taking a break of 4 to 7 days after every 2 weeks of treatment.

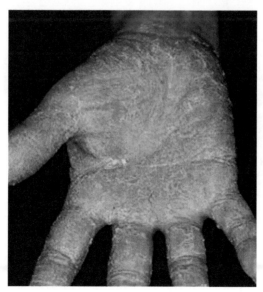

Fig. 3. Hand eczema. (*From* James WD, Berger TG, Elston DM. Andrews' diseases of the skin: clinical dermatology. Philadelphia: Saunders; 2016; with permission.)

Case 4

A 65-year-old woman with primary biliary cirrhosis presents with the nail examination shown in **Fig. 4**. Nail culture grows *Trichophyton rubrum*. She has tried ciclopirox on the nails nightly for 4 weeks without improvement. What treatment options are appropriate to discuss?

- Systemic treatment with terbinafine 250 mg daily for 6 weeks (fingernail treatment) or 12 weeks (toenail treatment) would not be recommended because the patient has known liver disease.
- The patient could continue ciclopirox for up to 48 weeks. Two double-blind, vehicle-controlled, parallel-group clinical trials show toenails with ~5.5% to 8.5% complete clinical clearance and 29% to 36% mycologic clearance after completing 48 weeks of treatment.[13] The patient may have not used the medication long enough to see a result. Fingernails take 6 months and toenails take 12 to 18 months to grow completely. It is important to counsel patients that they will not see immediate results with onychomycosis treatment whether or not they use topical or systemic therapy.

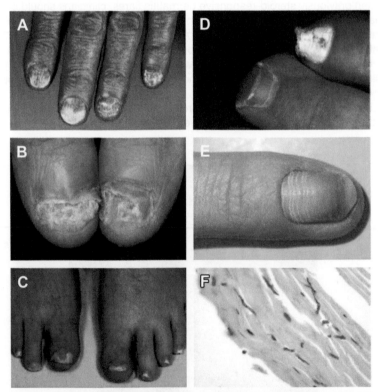

Fig. 4. Tinea unguium. Onycholysis, yellowing, crumbling, and thickening of the fingernails (*A*), thumb nails (*B*), and toenails (*C*) in the distal/lateral subungual variant. Diffuse (*D*) and striate (*E*) white discoloration of the toenail in the superficial white variant. Hyphae within formalin-fixed nail plate stained with periodic acid–Schiff (*F*). (*From* Elewski BE, Hughey LC, Sobera JO, et al. Fungal diseases. In: Bolognia J, Jorizzo JL, Schaffer JV, editors. Dermatology. Philadelphia: Elsevier Saunders; 2012; with permission.)

- She could switch to efinaconazole 10% solution and apply to the nails nightly for 48 weeks. Two recent phase III clinical trials show toenails with ~15% to 18% complete clinical clearance and 53% to 55% mycologic clearance 4 weeks after completing 48 weeks of treatment.[14] The efficacy of efinaconazole seems to be slightly greater than that of ciclopirox.

Case 5

A 66-year-old healthy man presents to clinic with yellow greasy scale with associated erythema and pruritus behind his ears, in his eyebrows, and on his scalp, as seen in **Fig. 5**. His wife is bothered by flakes falling on the patient's shirt and the cosmetic appearance. He is currently using his wife's shampoo because it smells good. What recommendations should be made?

- The patient has moderate seborrheic dermatitis, which is common, especially in the elderly and patients with neurologic conditions. He should discontinue his current shampoo and switch to either OTC antidandruff shampoo or prescription-strength ketoconazole 2% shampoo. Instruct the patient to let the shampoo sit on the scalp and face for 3 to 5 minutes before rinsing.
- A low-potency topical steroid (desonide 0.05% cream or hydrocortisone 2.5% cream), alone or mixed with ketoconazole 2% cream, can be applied behind ears and on eyebrows 1 to 2 times per day as needed to reduce redness and scaling.
- Despite his wife's concerns, if the patient is not bothered by the scaling, it could be argued that no treatment is necessary. Treatment of benign dermatoses such as seborrheic dermatitis is optional and many patients find using topical treatments cumbersome and unnecessary.

Case 6

An 18-year-old male teenager presents for follow up of acne shown in **Fig. 6**. He was last seen 4 weeks ago and was prescribed tretinoin 0.1% cream every night at bedtime, clindamycin 1% lotion every morning and an OTC benzoyl peroxide wash to use twice daily. He returns today because his skin is not improving and his acne medications are very irritating. What can be done to help?

- His follow-up appointment is too soon to evaluate the efficacy of his medications. If patients are tolerating their medications well, a follow-up in 2 to 3 months would be more appropriate. Acne medications take 6 to 8 weeks of regular use to see effect. It is important to emphasize that the tretinoin is to be used at night and applied to the entire face, not just on the individual acne lesions as spot treatment.
- His skin could be irritated for several reasons:
  - His tretinoin may be too strong. Options include decreasing the frequency of use to every other night, a trial of tretinoin 0.05% instead of 0.1%, or mixing a small amount of moisturizer with his current tretinoin cream to effectively dilute the concentration.
  - He may be using tretinoin immediately after washing his face or showering. Tretinoin can be very irritating if applied to a warm, flushed face. Instruct patient to wait 10 to 15 minutes after washing the face before applying tretinoin.
  - He may be irritated from using benzoyl peroxide twice daily. Advise him to use it only in the morning before he applies his topical clindamycin. He can use a gentle face cleanser in the evening.

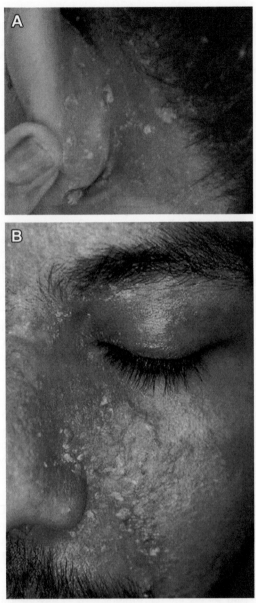

Fig. 5. Adult seborrheic dermatitis of the face, ear, and scalp. (*A*) Sharply demarcated pink plaque with white and greasy scale. Note the fissure in the retroauricular sulcus. (*B*) Sharply demarcated pink-orange thin plaques with yellow, greasy scale, especially in the melolabial fold. (*From* Reider N, Fritsch O. Other eczematous eruptions. In: Bolognia J, Jorizzo JL, Schaffer JV, editors. Dermatology. Philadelphia: Elsevier Saunders; 2012; with permission.)

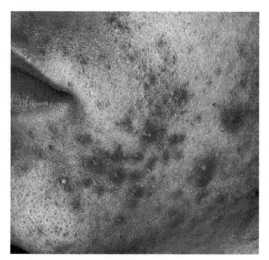

Fig. 6. Acne vulgaris, with papules and pustules, on the cheek. (*From* James WD, Berger TG, Elston DM. Andrews' diseases of the skin: clinical dermatology. Philadelphia: Saunders; 2016; with permission.)

SUMMARY

A representative assortment of topical therapies is discussed here with the goal of emphasizing the most commonly encountered diagnoses and treatments for nondermatologists. When using topical therapies, carefully consider the proper active ingredient, potency, vehicle, and quantity of medication. If topical therapy is ineffective, question whether the medication is being used properly, whether the diagnosis is correct, and whether the topical may be contributing to the problem. Examples of the topical contributing to the problem include tinea incognito exacerbated by topical steroid use and allergic contact dermatitis to topical steroid excipients. For some patients, even maximum topical therapy is insufficient and systemic treatment is required. At this point, consultation with a dermatologist may be helpful.

REFERENCES

1. Stern RS. The pattern of topical corticosteroid prescribing in the United States, 1989–1991. J Am Acad Dermatol 1996;35(2 Pt 1):183–6.
2. Sandoval LF, Davis SA, Feldman SR. Dermatologists' knowledge of and preferences regarding topical steroids. J Drugs Dermatol 2013;12(7):786–9.
3. Coondoo A, Phiske M, Verma S, et al. Side-effects of topical steroids: a long overdue revisit. Indian Dermatol Online J 2014;5(4):416–25.
4. Smack DP, Harrington AC, Dunn C, et al. Infection and allergy incidence in ambulatory surgery patients using white petrolatum vs bacitracin ointment. A randomized controlled trial. JAMA 1996;276(12):972–7.
5. Andriessen A, Lynde CW. Antibiotic resistance: shifting the paradigm in topical acne treatment. J Drugs Dermatol 2014;13(11):1358–64.
6. Swartzentruber GS, Yanta JH, Pizon AF. Methemoglobinemia as a complication of topical dapsone. N Engl J Med 2015;372(5):491–2.
7. Stein Gold L, Kircik L, Fowler J, et al. Long-term safety of ivermectin 1% cream vs azelaic acid 15% gel in treating inflammatory lesions of rosacea: results of two

40-week controlled, investigator-blinded trials. J Drugs Dermatol 2014;13(11): 1380–6.

8. Tanghetti EA, Jackson JM, Belasco KT, et al. Optimizing the use of topical brimonidine in rosacea management: panel recommendations. J Drugs Dermatol 2015; 14(1):33–40.

9. van Zuuren EJ, Kramer SF, Carter BR, et al. Effective and evidence-based management strategies for rosacea: summary of a Cochrane systematic review. Br J Dermatol 2011;165(4):760–81.

10. Micali G, Lacarrubba F, Nasca MR, et al. Topical pharmacotherapy for skin cancer: part I. Pharmacology. J Am Acad Dermatol 2014;70(6):965.e1–12 [quiz: 977–8].

11. Micali G, Lacarrubba F, Nasca MR, et al. Topical pharmacotherapy for skin cancer: part II. Clinical applications. J Am Acad Dermatol 2014;70(6):979.e1–12 [quiz: 9912].

12. Warshaw EM, Maibach HI, Taylor JS, et al. North American contact dermatitis group patch test results: 2011–2012. Dermatitis 2015;26(1):49–59.

13. Gupta AK, Fleckman P, Baran R. Ciclopirox nail lacquer topical solution 8% in the treatment of toenail onychomycosis. J Am Acad Dermatol 2000;43(4 Suppl): S70–80.

14. Elewski BE, Rich P, Pollak R, et al. Efinaconazole 10% solution in the treatment of toenail onychomycosis: two phase III multicenter, randomized, double-blind studies. J Am Acad Dermatol 2013;68(4):600–8.

Clinical Approach to Diffuse Blisters

Tarannum Jaleel, MD, Young Kwak, MD, Naveed Sami, MD*

KEYWORDS

- Blisters • Vesicles • Diffuse blisters • Vesiculobullous
- Autoimmune bullous disorders • Bullous drug eruptions

KEY POINTS

- A thorough history is essential because it may provide clues for both internal and external triggers of certain vesiculobullous eruptions. Medications are an important cause of bullous eruptions, which have the potential to be life threatening (eg, Stevens-Johnson syndrome/toxic epidermal necrolysis).
- Immunocompromised patients often have more severe and atypical manifestations of infectious vesiculobullous disease (eg, herpetic infections) and require more aggressive therapy.
- Specialized tests such as direct immunofluorescence and serologies are helpful in diagnosing certain autoimmune blistering diseases.
- Appropriate further testing should be considered because specific bullous eruptions are strongly associated with systemic diseases (eg, myeloproliferative disorders, connective tissue diseases, systemic vasculitides, inflammatory bowel disease, and certain infections).

At some point during their careers, it is likely that most physicians will encounter a patient who presents with blisters. The clinical presentation of vesicles and bullae suggests a broad differential and confusion often arises in how to approach such patients, especially if a dermatology service is not readily accessible. In most circumstances, these tend to be acute presentations. Although some blistering eruptions may be self-limited, others are life threatening, and prompt diagnosis and management are critical. This article (1) provides a systematic diagnostic approach to such patients, including history, physical examination, and relevant work-up (**Fig. 1**); and (2) introduces some common blistering diseases that may be encountered by primary care physicians and subspecialists.

This article originally appeared in Medical Clinics of North America, Volume 99, Issue 6, November 2015
Funding Sources: None.
Conflicts of Interest: None.
Department of Dermatology, University of Alabama at Birmingham, 1520 3rd Avenue South, EFH 414, Birmingham, AL 35294-0009, USA
* Corresponding author.
E-mail address: nsami@uab.edu

Physician Assist Clin 1 (2016) 307–331
http://dx.doi.org/10.1016/j.cpha.2015.12.007
2405-7991/16/$ – see front matter © 2016 Elsevier Inc. All rights reserved.

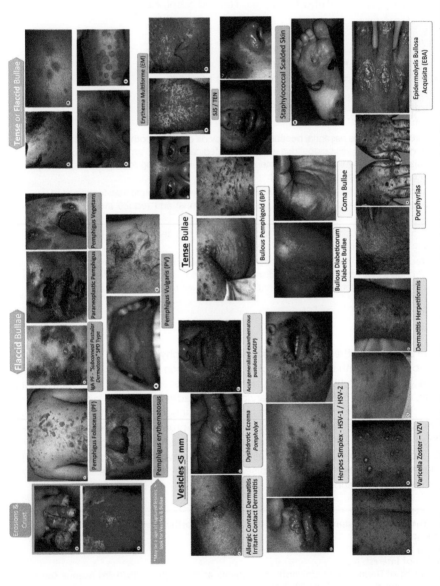

Fig. 1. Diagnostic approach for common vesiculobullous eruptions. Assoc., associated; IgA, immunoglobulin A; SJS, Stevens-Johnson syndrome; TEN, toxic epidermal necrolysis.

PATIENT HISTORY

During the initial encounter, a thorough history can play a vital role in determining the cause of a bullous eruption. There are many pertinent points in a history that help exclude possibilities, especially if the blistering eruption is atypical. Many of these variables are discussed here.

The age of onset can be crucial because certain bullous diseases are more common in specific age groups. Inherited blistering disorders such as epidermolysis bullosa begin in childhood, and may continue into adulthood.[1] Acquired processes such as autoimmune bullous disorders (ABDs) and bullous diseases secondary to systemic disease or external triggers can present in all age groups, but presentation may vary between children and adults.[2] For example, herpes zoster frequently presents in adults, whereas primary varicella presents more often in children.[3,4] Another example, staphylococcal scalded skin syndrome (SSSS), is more common in young children.

The timing of a rash can help identify acute causes, and tends to be related to particular triggers. Vesicles and bullae in the setting of external triggers, such as new medications, contact with chemicals/allergens, and infections, are acute in onset and tend to resolve after removal of the trigger. However, some ABDs and eruptions secondary to systemic disease are usually subacute to chronic with intermittent exacerbations and remissions.[2] As with any presenting illness, it is important to inquire about modifying factors that the patient may have observed in exacerbated and possibly accelerated progression of blisters. For example, photoaggravation of disease is seen in bullous lupus,[5] porphyria cutanea tarda,[6] and phytophotodermatitis,[7] whereas cold, wet environments worsen chilblains.[8]

A comprehensive review of systems is important because some diseases have particular prodromal symptoms that tend to continue as the blisters present and progress. Although diabetic bullae are asymptomatic,[9] bullous pemphigoid and contact dermatitis can be preceded by intense pruritus.[2,10] Necrotizing fasciitis and sepsis are frequent complications of bullous cellulitis associated with organisms like *Vibrio vulnificus*.[11] Immunosuppressed patients occasionally have atypical presentations, such as disseminated zoster.[3]

PHYSICAL EXAMINATION

Vesicles are elevated, fluid-filled, well-circumscribed clefts in the skin less than 1 cm in diameter, whereas bullae are greater than or equal to 1 cm in diameter (see **Fig. 1**). Although vesicles and bullae are the primary lesions, secondary changes such as crusting and erosions are concomitant in most blistering disorders. Herpes simplex and zoster, dyshidrotic eczema, and dermatitis herpetiformis present with a predominantly vesicular eruption, although in the dermatitis herpetiformis the eruption is often intensely itchy such that vesicles are excoriated before being recognized as blistering. Tense bullae (subepidermal split) are frequently seen in bullous pemphigoid, and flaccid bullae (intraepidermal split) in pemphigus vulgaris. Occasionally, only large erosions are present in cases of pemphigus foliaceous because the superficial bullae rupture before presentation. Nikolsky sign (shearing of epidermis with lateral pressure) is often seen with toxic epidermal necrolysis (TEN), SSSS, and pemphigus. Other commonly associated findings, such as erythematous urticarial plaques (eg, bullous pemphigoid), palpable purpura (eg, small vessel vasculitis), or targetoid macules (eg, erythema multiforme), can help facilitate a diagnosis.[12]

The configuration and pattern of blisters in a particular area can often provide clues to the diagnosis. Grouped vesicles are strongly suggestive of herpetic infections.[3] Geometric shapes and/or linear patterns are usually seen in the setting of phytophotodermatitis and contact dermatitis.[7,10] Annular configurations of bullae can suggest linear immunoglobulin (Ig) A bullous disease,[13] which is often described as resembling a string of pearls.

The area of distribution has important diagnostic implications, and includes the observation of key features such as the body areas involved (eg, acral/perioral/perineal), localized versus diffuse, photoexposed surfaces, and mucosal or conjunctival involvement. Localized distributions are seen in herpes zoster (dermatomal),[3] porphyria cutanea tarda (hands),[6] phototoxic drug eruptions (face, neck, and dorsal arms),[14] and diabetic bullae (areas of trauma, typically shins).[9,14] Mucosal involvement is seen in pemphigus and some variants of pemphigoid.[15,16]

DIAGNOSTIC TESTING

Initial diagnostic testing is ordered based on history and physical examination. In acute settings, diagnosis often relies on a bedside clinical assessment. If there are multiple possibilities, a skin (punch) biopsy of a new vesicle or the edge of an intact blister is recommended. Direct immunofluorescence (DIF) testing of a biopsy from perilesional skin along with serologic testing for relevant antibodies is helpful in differentiating various autoimmune bullous diseases. Special stains for infections can also be performed on biopsies. However, swabbing the skin for cultures and viral polymerase chain reaction (PCR) is easier, faster, and may provide more information. Additional pertinent blood tests can be performed based on the initial results to help identify any systemic causes.[12]

BLISTERING CONDITIONS CAUSED BY EXTERNAL TRIGGERS
Allergic Contact Dermatitis

Background
Allergic contact dermatitis (ACD) is the result of a type IV, delayed type, hypersensitivity response to specific allergens in the setting of prior sensitization. Subsequent reexposure to an allergen at low concentrations is often sufficient to elicit a response.[10,17,18]

History
Patients with ACD present with significant pruritus accompanying a rash, which usually develops within days of exposure to a specific allergen. It is important to inquire about changes to a patient's daily routine, including new hobbies or occupations, or the recent use of new products. Location of the rash may help determine the cause. For example, a rash around the neck and earlobes may indicate an allergy to nickel, which is present in some jewelry. A detailed history can help identify the cause of less common presentations such as eyelid dermatitis, which may be caused by a new nail polish.[10,17,18]

Physical examination
ACD typically presents as a well-demarcated pruritic eruption. Blisters and vesicles are often seen in an acute setting, whereas eczematous erythematous patches and plaques are more typical in the chronic setting. Geometric configurations, such as linear streaks caused by poison ivy dermatitis, are a key examination clue to ACD. Diffuse patchy eruptions well away from the primary contact reaction may be associated with autosensitization (the so-called id reaction). Occasionally, ACD and systemic autosensitization may result in erythroderma.[10,17,18]

Differential diagnosis
Irritant contact dermatitis (discussed later), dyshidrotic eczema, and bullous tinea pedis. Erythroderma that is caused by mycosis fungoides, medications, or other causes.

Diagnostic study/biopsy
ACD is generally diagnosed by history and physical examination. In some cases, a biopsy may help exclude other diagnoses. The histology usually shows spongiotic dermatitis with a mixed inflammatory infiltrate including eosinophils. Patch testing is the gold standard to identify an allergen. The top 10 common allergens are presented in **Table 1**.[10,17,18]

Treatment
The primary treatment is avoidance of the allergen, and provision of information regarding products containing identified allergens. It may take several weeks for the eruption to resolve despite allergen avoidance. Medium-potency to high-potency topical steroids may be used in localized cases. A systemic corticosteroid taper over 2 to 3 weeks may be indicated in severe cases. This treatment is typically reserved for contact dermatitis involving involvement of body surface areas of greater than 20%.[10,18]

Irritant Contact Dermatitis

Background
Irritant contact dermatitis (ICD) results from a local caustic reaction to chemicals. Chronic repetitive exposure to various mild irritants, such as soaps and cleansers, leads to breakdown of the skin barrier, and can present with various morphologies ranging from erythema and scaling to vesicles and bullae.[19,20]

History
Onset often is not abrupt, and the condition is usually chronic with intermittent flares. Affected areas tend to be painful rather than pruritic. Patients usually have a history of repetitive chronic exposure to low-grade irritants such as soaps and solvents. Bullae are more likely with exposure to strong irritants such as alkali or acids.[20]

Physical examination
Patients usually present with well-defined vesicular, bullous, or scaly erythematous patches corresponding with sites of contact. For example, ICD of the hands frequently presents with vesicles and scaly erythematous patches on the lateral aspects of

Table 1
Top 10 allergens as identified by the North American Contact Dermatitis Group

Test Substance	Allergic Reactions (%)	Relevant Reactions: Definite, Probable, Possible Combined (%)
Nickel sulfate	19	57
Myroxylon pereirae (balsam of Peru)	12	87
Fragrance mix 1	11.5	86
Quaternium-15	10	89
Neomycin sulfate	10	28
Bacitracin	9	39
Formaldehyde	9	91
Cobalt chloride	8.5	48
Methyldibromoglutaronitrile/ phenoxyethanol	6	75
p-Phenylenediamine	5	56

From Mowad CM, Marks JG. Allergic contact dermatitis. In: Bolognia JL, Jorizzo JL, Schaeffer JV, editors. Dermatology. London: Saunders; 2012; with permission.

fingers in the setting of chronic exposure to soaps and cleansers. Prolonged contact with irritants may eventually cause thickening of skin and fissuring. Involved areas can be painful and thus limit activity.[20] ACD to leather gloves can have similar appearance with localized lesions at sites of contact.[14]

Differential diagnosis
Excluding ACD can be difficult without patch testing. Also consider tinea manuum or pustular psoriasis with localized lesions on the hands. Dyshidrotic eczema (pompholyx) is a chronic and recurrent palmoplantar dermatosis with a similar clinical appearance, and is a result of atopic dermatitis with a component of ICD and/or ACD.[7,20] However, this entity is a diagnosis of exclusion and external triggers must be addressed.

Diagnostic study/biopsy
Diagnosis is based on clinical history. Biopsy can be helpful but is not definitive, and usually shows a spongiotic dermatitis with occasional necrotic keratinocytes and a lymphocytic infiltrate.[19]

Treatment/further work-up
The focus of treatment is the restoration of the skin barrier and removal of the trigger. In general, topical steroids, barrier creams, and avoidance of irritants are critical in management. Treatments in the setting of exposure to alkali or acid products are agent dependent.[19]

Phototoxic Bullous Eruption (Phytophotodermatitis)

Background
Phototoxic bullous eruptions are caused by contact with agents containing furocoumarins. Furocoumarins are toxic to skin on conversion by ultraviolet (UV) light. Phytophotodermatitis is a result of UV exposure to plant sources of furocoumarins.[7,21]

History and physical examination
The eruption begins 30 minutes to 2 hours after UV exposure and progresses to burning, erythema, vesicles, and blisters over the following 2 to 3 days. The clinical appearance is distinctive, with vesicles in a linear or geometric pattern, and bulla with concomitant erythema. The rash usually resolves with hyperpigmentation that can persist for several months. Of note, some cases show recurrence in the identical site on exposure to UV several months after the initial presentation. Patients may present at any stage, and diagnosis may be difficult when asymptomatic or with only residual hyperpigmentation. It is important to obtain a history regarding exposures within 2 to 3 days before initial presentation to plants (ie, celery, lime, or rue), medications (application of insect repellants or consumption of psoralens), and fragrances containing bergamot compounds.[7,21]

Differential diagnosis
Photoallergic contact dermatitis, bullous lupus, porphyria cutanea tarda, photoallergic drug-induced photosensitivity, and pseudoporphyria.

Diagnostic study/biopsy
A biopsy can be helpful when the diagnosis is unclear, and usually shows epidermal hyperkeratosis, spongiosis with necrotic keratinocytes, and occasionally intraepidermal and subepidermal blistering. The inflammatory infiltrate can vary with neutrophils and a perivascular lymphohistiocytic infiltrate with occasional eosinophils (in the acute setting). Later stages may show melanophages with pigment incontinence, increased melanin, melanocytic hyperplasia with variable acanthosis, hyperkeratosis, and hypergranulosis.[7,21]

Treatment/further work-up

Treatment in the acute setting depends on the severity of involvement. Topical steroids with antihistamines can be considered initially. Oral corticosteroids may be required for severe involvement. Strict, long-term sun avoidance is also necessary to avoid flares.[7,21]

Bullous Arthropod Bite Reactions

Background

An exaggerated bite response to mosquitoes, fleas, scabies, and bed bugs can sometimes be seen in children or in individuals with myeloproliferative disorders such as chronic lymphocytic leukemia.[14,22]

History

Patients present with an acute onset of blisters associated with intense pruritus localized to the affected site. Patients may not always recall a history of bug bites, but they have usually been outdoors.[14,22]

Physical examination

Bites usually present as grouped pink papules, but in some cases progress to vesicles or blisters. In cases associated with hematological malignancies, large bullae and necrosis can be seen (**Fig. 2**).[14,22]

Differential diagnosis

Bullous impetigo, bullous erythema multiforme, bullous Sweet syndrome, and localized ABDs such as bullous pemphigoid.

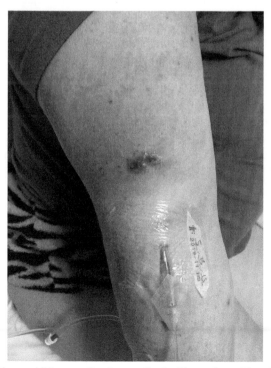

Fig. 2. Bullous arthropod bite eruption in a patient with myeloproliferative disorder.

Diagnostic study/biopsy
Biopsy shows a superficial and deep perivascular infiltrate with eosinophils along with possible epidermal necrosis at the bite site. Eosinophilic spongiosis is seen in the early phase, and may progress to subepidermal blisters.[14,22]

Treatment
Supportive care with antihistamines and topical corticosteroids for symptomatic control. Consider systemic corticosteroids if previous treatments are not sufficient. Counsel on insect avoidance and the use of insect repellants and protective clothing.[14,22]

AUTOIMMUNE BULLOUS DISORDERS

ABDs are a group of diseases with autoantibody formation to various components of the epidermis and basement membrane.[5] For example, autoantibodies targeting desmosomes in the epidermis result in an intraepidermal split presenting as flaccid bullae and erosions (mucosal and skin), as seen in pemphigus (see **Fig. 1**). Autoantibodies against hemidesmosomes and other components of the basement membrane zone result in a subepidermal split leading to disorders including pemphigoid, as detailed in **Table 2**.[1,2,12,15,16,23–25] Diagnosis requires a combination of clinical, histopathologic, immunofluorescence, and serologic findings. In performing a skin biopsy, a well-developed new vesicle or the edge of an intact blister should be sampled. The level of split, along with concomitant histologic findings, is essential to the diagnosis. DIF evaluation of perilesional skin is helpful in differentiating an ABD from a non-ABD and between various ABDs. In some cases, such as dermatitis herpetiformis, sampling of normal skin directly adjacent to vesicles and bullae is necessary in order to detect sufficient antibodies to make the diagnosis. Special stains can also be used to detect organisms. Various serologic tests are also commercially available to confirm the diagnosis of various ABDs (see **Table 2**). Appropriate early treatment and management are critical given the significant disease morbidity and mortality.[12]

BULLOUS ERUPTIONS ASSOCIATED WITH INTERNAL DISEASES
Bullous Diabeticorum

Background
Diabetic patients can develop bullae on distal extremities, most commonly at sites of trauma. Although the cause is unclear, these bullae are exacerbated by concomitant microangiopathy.[9,14]

History
Blisters are sudden in onset and generally asymptomatic, but patients may experience a prodrome of burning in the affected area before onset. Patients tend to have other diabetic complications, such as diabetic neuropathy and systemic organ involvement (ie, nephropathy, retinopathy).[9,14]

Physical examination
Tense bullae are typically distributed on the distal extremities (most commonly feet and legs), and usually have no surrounding inflammation or erythema. The fluid within the bullae is usually clear and viscous in consistency.[9,14]

Differential diagnosis
Friction blisters, pseudoporphyria, bullous pemphigoid, and edema bullae.

Table 2
Autoimmune bullous diseases: clinical characteristics, work-up, and management

Disease	Level of Split	Clinical Characteristics	DDX	Work-up	Treatment
Pemphigus: • PV • PF • Other subtypes (see **Fig. 1**)	Intraepidermal (suprabasal)	• Mean age of onset usually 50–60 y, but may affect all ages • Present with painful erosions and flaccid bullae, most commonly on torso • Tend to heal slowly with hyperpigmentation • Pruritus less common • PF: may have only erosions and crusts • PV: oral mucosa is most commonly affected and predominant finding is painful erosions • PV may involve other mucosal surfaces (conjunctiva, pharynx, larynx, esophagus, nasal, anal, genital) • Other symptoms: hoarseness and dysphagia • Clinical course: chronic with intermittent flares	• Acute herpetic flare, EM, SJS • Mucosal forms of pemphigoid may present with similar mucosal erosions and blisters • Consider paraneoplastic pemphigus in recalcitrant cases	• H&E: Intraepidermal acantholysis • DIF: perilesional skin with antibodies to keratinocyte cell surface • IIF and ELISA: IgG autoantibodies against DSG 1 and 3 correlate with disease activity • PF: autoantibodies to DSG1 (predominantly skin) • PV: autoantibodies to DSG3 (predominantly mucosal) ± DSG1 (skin)	• Prompt treatment is critical because it is potentially fatal • Initial treatment: systemic corticosteroids with slow transition to steroid-sparing agents to minimize adverse effects of corticosteroids • Supportive measures during flares: pain management, nonadherent dressings, topical steroids • Some commonly used steroid-sparing agents: azathioprine, MMF, cyclophosphamide, MTX, IVIg, rituximab, plasmapheresis

(continued on next page)

Table 2
(continued)

Disease	Level of Split	Clinical Characteristics	DDX	Work-up	Treatment
BP	Supepidermal (hemidesmosome)	• Typically affects the elderly • Very pruritic • Rarely with pain in oral cavity, dysphagia, or dysuria secondary to mucosal involvement • Diverse skin manifestations: before progressing to bullae formation, may present with pruritus and no skin lesions, excoriations, erythematous eczematous plaques, and/or urticarial erythematous plaques • Some patients may present only with urticarial plaques with excoriations • Although mucosal involvement is rare, erosions and ulcers can involve the oral cavity and genitalia • Lesions distributed symmetrically predominantly on lower trunk and lower extremities • Clinical course: chronic with frequent exacerbations and remissions	• Nonbullous phase: urticaria, urticarial vasculitis • Bullous phase: EBA, bullous lupus, LABD, drug-induced, bullous EM, bullous bite reaction, edema bullae, bullous diabeticorum	• H&E: bullous phase, subepidermal blister with predominant eosinophils in a mixed inflammatory infiltrate • H&E: nonbullous phase, subepidermal cleft + epidermal spongiosis and/or dermal eosinophils • DIF: Perilesional skin shows antibodies against epidermal basement membrane (hemidesmosome components) • Salt-split skin[a]: IgG autoantibodies bind to epidermal side of blister • Commercial ELISA serologic tests are available to check for autoantibodies to BP antigens (180 and 230)	• Potent topical steroids: useful in mild and moderate nonprogressive disease • Systemic steroids: initial mainstay of treatment of severe progressive disease • Chronic systemic treatment can vary depending on severity of disease and comorbidities. These can include tetracyclines (± nicotinamide), dapsone, azathioprine, MTX, MMF, rituximab
Bullous lupus	Subepidermal (sub–lamina densa)	• Female predilection, affecting individuals aged 20–40 y • Acute onset and can be the first sign of SLE • Can be accompanied by other systemic manifestations of SLE	• Subepidermal ABDs (BP, inflammatory EBA) • Phototoxic drug reactions • PCT	• H&E: lesional skin from intact blister shows subepidermal blister with neutrophils • DIF: granular deposition of autoantibodies along the BMZ	• Dapsone along with other immunosuppressants • Rituximab has been used with some success in recalcitrant cases

| | | • Often presents in the spring and summer with more sun exposure
• Vesicles and bullae develop within existing lupus lesions or de novo with predilection for sun-exposed areas such as face, trunk, and arms
• Lesions tend to heal with no scarring or milia | • Can be mistaken for SJS/TEN if involvement is extensive and leading to desquamation | • Serologies: autoantibodies to type 7 collagen, ANA, anti-dsDNA, anti-Sm, anti-Ro/SS-A, anti-La/SS-B | |
| EBA | Subepidermal (sub–lamina densa) | • Rare chronic condition with slow onset affecting trauma-prone skin and mucous membranes
• Can occur at any age
• Has been associated with inflammatory bowel disease
• Presents with tense bullae on trauma-prone sites (eg, knuckles, wrists, extensor surfaces, hands and feet) and tend to heal with milia, and scarring
• Scarring alopecia may develop with scalp involvement
• Inflammatory subtype of EBA tends to be more acute and generalized, and blisters may also involve flexural as well as intertriginous areas
• Mucosal involvement: oral, nasal, conjunctival, laryngeal, pharyngeal, esophageal, urogenital, anal
• Mucosal lesions can lead to irreversible scarring and dysfunction | • ABDs: BP, LABD, bullous lupus | • H&E: subepidermal blister with a mixed inflammatory infiltrate
• DIF: autoantibody IgG along the BMZ in a U-serrated pattern
• Salt-split skin[a]: autoantibody binding to the dermal side of the salt-split skin
• ELISA: detect autoantibodies to type VII collagen
• Age-specific cancer screening recommended | • Systemic corticosteroids, dapsone, colchicine, and other conventional immunosuppressants |

(continued on next page)

Table 2
(continued)

Disease	Level of Split	Clinical Characteristics	DDX	Work-up	Treatment
Pemphigoid gestationis	Subepidermal	• Rare pruritic blistering condition seen in late pregnancy or early postpartum • Present acutely with pruritic urticarial plaques progressing to grouped vesicles and tense bullae • May be present predominantly around the umbilicus/abdomen, and can progress to involve the entire body, especially around the time of delivery • Concurrent erythematous plaques and papules are also present • Occasionally, the neonate has vesicles and blisters caused by maternal transfer of antibodies (IgG) • Most cases resolve a few weeks after delivery, but may flare around menstruation, with use of oral contraceptives, or with recurrent pregnancies • Associated with an increased risk of Graves disease and antithyroid antibodies may be present on evaluation • Precautions should be taken because of a higher risk of prematurity and small-for-gestational-age size	• PEP/PUPPP • Urticaria	• H&E: subepidermal vesicle with eosinophils on lesional skin • DIF: most commonly shows C3 deposition along the BMZ • Monitor newborn for bullae	• Topical corticosteroids + antihistamines (category B) for minor disease • Oral corticosteroids for severe disease • Unusual for disease to persist after delivery • Provide counseling because the disease may flare with oral contraceptives and subsequent pregnancies

| Dermatitis herpetiformis | Subepidermal | • Seen in genetically predisposed individuals with gluten sensitivity and most patients have some form of gastrointestinal involvement (celiac disease)
• Chronic, lifelong condition with intermittent flares and remissions correlating with gluten consumption. Spontaneous remission is rare
• Significant pruritus
• Diarrhea and abdominal pain may be present in patients with celiac disease
• Symmetrically distributed grouped erythematous papules, vesicles, and plaques with surrounding erythema most commonly on extensor surfaces (dorsal forearms, elbows, knees), buttocks, and back
• Secondary excoriations and hemorrhagic crusting also present in most cases caused by severe pruritus | • ABDs: LABD, EBA, BP
• Infections (herpetic)
• Drug-induced blisters
• Folliculitis
• Pityriasis lichenoides | • H&E: biopsy of a vesicle with a subepidermal blister and predominant neutrophils along the dermal papillae
• DIF: uninvolved adjacent skin shows granular autoantibody IgA deposition along the dermal papillae
• Serologies: positive for antiendomysial and antitransglutaminase (tissue and epidermal) autoantibodies
• May be associated with other autoimmune diseases; consider monitoring of blood glucose and thyroid function
• Referral to gastroenterology for celiac disease and surveillance for lymphoma | • Significant improvement can be seen with avoidance of gluten and use of dapsone |

Abbreviations: ANA, antinuclear antibodies; anti-Sm, anti-Smith; Anti-SSA, Anti-Sjogren's Syndrome A; Anti-SSB, Anti-Sjogren's Syndrome B; BMZ, basement membrane zone; BP, bullous pemphigoid; C3, complement 3; DDX, differential diagnosis; DIF, direct immunofluorescence; dsDNA, double-stranded DNA; DSG, desmoglein; EBA, epidermolysis bullosa acquisita; ELISA, enzyme-linked immunosorbent assay; EM, erythema multiforme; H&E, hematoxylin and eosin; IVIg, intravenous immunoglobulin; La, Anti-SSB; LABD, linear IgA bullous disease (see text); IgA, immunoglobulin A; IgG, immunoglobulin G; IIF, indirect Immunofluorescence; MMF, mycophenolate mofetil; MTX, methotrexate; PCT, porphyria cutanea tarda; PEP, polymorphic eruption of pregnancy; PF, pemphigus foliaceus; PUPPP, pruritic urticarial papules and plaques of pregnancy; PV, pemphigus vulgaris; Ro, Anti-SSA; SJS, Stevens-Johnson syndrome; SLE, systemic lupus erythematosus; TEN, toxic epidermal necrolysis.

^a Specimens incubated in 5 mL of NaCl (1 mol/L) at 4°C for 24 hours. Epidermis then separated from dermis and specimens processed in same manner and treated with IgG and C3 conjugates as in DIF. BP shows floor pattern and EBA shows roof pattern; correlates with autoantibodies against hemidesmosomal proteins versus collagen 7, respectively.

Diagnostic study/biopsy

Biopsy shows primarily subepidermal blisters in active lesions, and intraepidermal splits in older lesions. Friction blisters show a split below the stratum granulosum and are usually seen in the setting of repetitive trauma. DIF is negative.[9,14]

Treatment

Supportive care, treatment with an aluminum acetate solution, and prevention of infection.[9,14]

Chilblains

Background

Chilblains occur with exposure of acral surfaces (hands and feet) to cold, wet environments. It is an aberrant response in predisposed individuals, and has an unknown pathogenesis.[8,26]

History

Chilblains are commonly seen in women, children, and elderly living in cold climates with no central heating. It is a chronic condition affecting acral surfaces, and may involve the ears and nose. There is usually an associated burning pain and occasionally pruritus.[8,26]

Physical examination

The eruptions usually present as violaceous to erythematous macules, papules, or patches on volar surfaces of the distal toes and fingers, ears, and nose. Severe cases may progress to blistering and ulceration.[8,26]

Differential diagnosis

Cryoglobulinemia, myelomonocytic leukemia, hemolytic anemia, chilblain lupus erythematosus, Raynaud phenomenon, and several other cold-induced eruptions should be considered. Second-degree and third-degree frostbite also have a similar acral distribution with bullae.[8,26]

Diagnostic study/biopsy

Biopsy shows papillary dermal edema with a superficial and deep lymphocytic infiltrate, and can be helpful in distinguishing from other entities, such as chilblain lupus. Laboratory evaluation is necessary to rule out systemic causes.[8,26]

Treatment

Calcium channel blockers (amlodipine and nifedipine), cold weather clothing, and avoidance of cold and wet environments are recommended. Hydroxychloroquine can be considered if associated with systemic lupus erythematosus.[8,26]

Coma Bullae

Background

Coma bullae were previously referred to as barbiturate bullae. Although the exact cause is unknown, they are frequently seen with prolonged immobilization caused by loss of consciousness (ie, neurologic and endocrine disorders, medications, illicit drug use),[14,27] thus pressure-induced injury may play a role in pathogenesis.

History

Blisters generally develop acutely at sites of greatest pressure within 48 to 72 hours of loss of consciousness, and tend to be asymptomatic.[14,27]

Physical examination

Tense blisters develop over bony prominences and areas of greatest pressure, and eventually result in erosions.[14,27]

Differential diagnosis

Bullous diabeticorum and friction blisters.

Diagnostic study/biopsy

Biopsy shows a subepidermal split along with eccrine sweat gland necrosis, which helps to distinguish coma bullae from other blistering entities. Additional findings of rhabdomyolysis and compression neuropathy may be seen in some patients.[14,27]

Treatment

Avoidance of pressure to sites with bullae to prevent further progression, supportive wound care, toxicology evaluation, and review of medications.[14,27]

Edema Bullae

Background

Edema bullae develop because of sudden acute swelling in patients with underlying comorbidities such as congestive heart failure, renal disease, liver disease, or thrombosis leading to lower extremity edema and/or anasarca.[12,14]

History

Bullae usually develop acutely and are asymptomatic. In patients with conditions leading to chronic fluid overload, acute exacerbations can cause increased edema of the lower extremities that may be painful.[14,27]

Physical examination

Tense bullae with clear to serosanguineous fluid and minimal surrounding inflammation as well as concomitant edema are usually seen. This condition predominantly occurs in acutely ill hospitalized patients receiving excessive intravenous fluids, or in the setting of anasarca. Bullae may be localized to the distal lower extremities (dorsal foot and ankle) in patients with heart or kidney disease who acutely develop increased swelling from baseline.[14,27]

Differential diagnosis

Bullous diabeticorum, bullous pemphigoid, and medication-induced bullous eruptions, including drug-induced ABDs (discussed later).

Diagnostic study/biopsy

Biopsy usually shows a very edematous dermis with splayed collagen bundles, significant epidermal spongiosis, and occasionally subepidermal bullae.[14,27]

Treatment

Usually resolves with resolution of edema and, generally, no additional treatment is necessary.[14,27]

Porphyria Cutanea Tarda

Background

Porphyrias are a group of disorders resulting from acquired or inherited defects in the enzymes responsible for heme synthesis. Porphyria cutanea tarda results from decreased activity of uroporphyrinogen decarboxylase[6,10] and is the most common porphyria presenting in an adult population. Iron overload plays an integral part in its pathogenesis.

History

The initial symptoms include photosensitivity along with skin breakdown, and are usually precipitated by a variety of risk factors, such as alcohol consumption, increased estrogen levels, increased iron levels (as seen in hemochromatosis), hepatitis C, and human immunodeficiency virus (HIV).[6,10] Lesions are typically very slow to heal.

Physical examination

Minimal trauma leads to blistering and erosions with overlying crust symmetrically distributed on photoexposed skin (especially the face and dorsal hands). These areas heal with postinflammatory pigmentary alterations. Milia and waxy, yellow, plaquelike scarring may develop. In rare cases, contractures of the digits may occur. Patients may also have a unique finding of increased hair on the bitemporal and malar cheeks. In some cases, permanent loss of scalp hair and fingernails can be seen. Urine is usually slightly brown or discolored.[6,10]

Differential diagnosis

Drug-induced bullae, pseudoporphyria (**Table 3**), and ABDs (BP, epidermolysis bullosa acquisita, bullous lupus) (see **Table 2**).

Diagnostic study/biopsy

Diagnosis is confirmed with laboratory abnormalities showing increased serum and urine uroporphyrin, urine coproporphyrin, and fecal isocoproporphyrin. Further evaluation should include tests for hepatitis C, HIV, hemochromatosis, hemoglobin/hematocrit, liver function, and iron studies (particularly ferritin). Biopsy is not always necessary because the condition is fairly recognizable based on clinical appearance and laboratory testing.[6,10]

Treatment/further work-up

Initially consider serial phlebotomies every 2–4 weeks with monitoring of hemoglobin, hematocrit, and iron levels with the goal to reach a hemoglobin level of 10 to 11 g/dL and the lower limits of normal range of serum ferritin concentration without induction of iron deficiency anemia. Low-dose antimalarials (ie, hydroxychloroquine 100 mg twice weekly) have also been successful. Erythropoietin has been reported to be helpful in patients with renal failure. Photoprotection, avoidance of triggers such as alcohol, and treatment of associated conditions are also recommended. It is important to monitor for the development of hepatocellular carcinoma given the increased long-term risk in these patients.[6,10]

Bullous Neutrophilic Dermatoses

Background

Bullous neutrophilic dermatoses are inflammatory dermatoses with 2 major subtypes: bullous Sweet syndrome (BSS) and bullous pyoderma gangrenosum (BPG). There has been a suggestion that BSS and BPG are variants of the same disease process.[28]

History

BPG presents with painful blisters that are acute in onset and rapidly progressive. BPG has been seen in association with systemic diseases, including hematologic malignancies and inflammatory bowel disease.[28] Sweet syndrome usually presents with fever, an increased neutrophil count, and joint involvement, and may be associated with myelogenous leukemia, medications, autoimmune disorders, and infections.[29]

Physical examination

BPG presents as flaccid hemorrhagic bullae sometimes overlying an erythematous plaque, and progresses to superficial ulcerations most commonly on the face and

Table 3
Bullous drug eruptions

Disease	Examination Findings	Time Interval	Notes	Notable Responsible Drugs	Treatment
Fixed drug eruption	• Sharply circumscribed erythematous to dusky violaceous patches • Central blisters or erosions may appear • Often resolves with postinflammatory hyperpigmentation • Recurrence at same locations following drug reexposure • Can involve mucosa and genitalia	• First exposure, 1–2 wk • Reexposure, <48 h, usually within 24 h	• May have mucosal, acral, and genital involvement	Sulfonamides, TMP-SMX, NSAIDs, aspirin, acetaminophen (paracetamol), barbiturates, phenolphthalein, tetracyclines, metronidazole, pseudoephedrine	—

SJS TEN	• Prodromal symptoms: fever and painful skin
	• Dusky macules with or without epidermal detachment
	• Macular atypical targets
	• Flaccid bullous lesions, confluence, wide erosions + Nikolsky sign
	• Involves mucosa, face, trunk
	• Systemic symptoms: fever, lymphadenopathy, hepatitis, and cytopenias
		7–21 d	• Mucosal, acral, and genital involvement
			• Percentage detachment of BSA
			  ○ SJS <10%
			  ○ SJS-TEN overlap 10%–30%
			  ○ TEN >30%
				Sulfonamides, TMP-SMX, allopurinol, β-lactam Abx, NSAIDs, piroxicam, anticonvulsants (aromatic), lamotrigine, phenytoin, barbiturates	• Critical = early withdrawal of responsible drug
					• No definitive therapy
					• Supportive care with burn team
					• Corticosteroids controversial
					• IVIg, cyclosporine, cyclophosphamide, plasmapheresis, N-acetylcysteine, TNF-α antagonists

(continued on next page)

Table 3
(continued)

Disease	Examination Findings	Time Interval	Notes	Notable Responsible Drugs	Treatment
EM	• Rarely drug induced, ~90% from infections (HSV-1/2, *Myco-plasma pneumoniae*, VZV, EBV, CMV, *Histoplasma capsulatum*, dermatophytes, and so forth) • Targetoid lesions on extremities/face • EM minor: target lesions, papular atypical targets, possible mucosal involvement. No systemic symptoms • EM major: as above + severe mucosal involvement, systemic symptoms, may have bullous lesions	—	• Rarely drug induced • Mostly from infections • No progression to TEN	NSAIDs, sulfonamides, anticonvulsants, aminopenicillins, allopurinol	• Consider prophylaxis for recurrent disease (acyclovir/valacyclovir/famciclovir) • Early systemic corticosteroids or pulse methylprednisolone may help • Refractory disease: azathioprine, thalidomide, dapsone, cyclosporine, mycophenolate mofetil, PUVA
AGEP	• Acute onset with high fever • Usually occurs within 2 d of drug exposure • Areas of erythema studded with pustules and occasionally vesicles • Lesions begin on face or intertriginous areas	<4 d	• High fever • Malaise, leukocytosis • >90% of cases drug induced	β-Lactams, macrolides, pristinamycin, terbinafine, hydroxychloroquine, calcium channel blockers (diltiazem), carbamazepine, acetaminophen, metronidazole	• Withdrawal of responsible drug • Topical corticosteroids • Antipyretics
Phototoxic drug eruption	• Limited to sun-exposed areas • Resembles exaggerated sunburn	—	—	Tetracyclines (especially doxycycline), quinolones, psoralens, NSAIDs, diuretics	—

	Clinical features		Associated features	Causative drugs	Treatment
Drug-induced linear IgA bullous dermatosis	• Circumferential and linear vesicles and bullae • Annular and herpetiform vesicopustules and plaques	—	—	Vancomycin most common, β-lactam Abx, captopril, NSAIDs	• Topical steroids and withdrawal of drug usually lead to improvement • Systemic steroids and SSTs can be considered for patients with chronic disease
Drug-induced PV	• Most develop painful oral erosions • Flaccid blisters • Widespread cutaneous erosions • Associated pruritus uncommon (unlike bullous pemphigoid)	—	• Mucosal involvement • Paraneoplastic pemphigus has severe stomatitis/mucosal erosions	• 80% caused by drugs with a thiol group: penicillamine, ACE inhibitors (captopril), gold sodium thiomalate, pyritinol • Nonthiol drugs: antibiotics (especially β-lactams), pyrazolone derivatives, nifedipine, propranolol, piroxicam, and phenobarbital	• Mainstay = systemic corticosteroids • Topical = corticosteroids, antibiotics, immunomodulators (eg, tacrolimus) • If unresolved after medication withdrawal and corticosteroids, similar to pemphigus (see **Table 2**)
Drug-induced bullous pemphigoid	• Most common autoimmune subepidermal blistering disease • Associated with severe pruritus • Tense bullae on normal and erythematous skin • Concomitant erythematous or urticarial plaques	—	• May have mucosal, acral, and genital involvement • Predominantly elderly • May be preceded by a pruritic urticarial or exanthematous phase	Furosemide, penicillin and other β-lactams, sulfasalazine	• Mainstay = systemic corticosteroids • Topical = corticosteroids, antibiotics, immunomodulators (eg, tacrolimus) • If unresolved after medication withdrawal and corticosteroids, consider SSTs (see **Table 2**)
Drug-induced pseudoporphyria	• Resembles PCT • Porphyrins are within normal limits	—	• Sun-exposed surfaces	NSAIDs (naproxen), nalidixic acid, thiazides, furosemide, tetracyclines	Withdrawal of responsible drug

Abbreviations: Abx, antibiotics; ACE, angiotensin-converting enzyme; AGEP, acute generalized exanthematous pustulosis; BSA, body surface area; CMV, cytomegalovirus; d, days; EBV, Epstein-Barr virus; h, hours; EM, erythema multiforme; HSV, herpes simplex virus; IVIG, intravenous immunoglobulins; NSAID, nonsteroidal antiinflammatory drug; PCT, porphyria cutanea tarda; PUVA, psoralen (P) and ultraviolet A (UVA) therapy; PV, pemphigus vulgaris; SJS, stevens johnson syndrome; SSTs, steroid-sparing treatments; TEN, toxic epidermis necrolysis wk, week(s); TMP-SMX trimethoprim-sulfamethoxazole; TNF-α, tumor necrosis factor alpha; VZV, varicella zoster Virus.

Adapted from Bolognia JL, Jorizzo JL, Schaeffer JV, editors. Dermatology. London: Saunders; 2012.

upper extremities.[28] The typical lesions of Sweet syndrome are edematous, translucent, and erythematous papules and plaques that tend to localize to the head, neck, trunk, and upper extremities, but can also be widespread. Oral involvement may be seen in cases associated with hematologic malignancies. In BSS, vesicles containing viscous fluid can occasionally proceed to ulceration.[29]

Differential diagnosis
V vulnificus, leishmaniasis, and exaggerated bite reactions.

Diagnostic study/biopsy
Biopsies of both processes show a neutrophilic dermal infiltrate. Papillary dermal edema is prominent in BSS, and a subepidermal split is seen in BPG. A thorough history, review of medications, and evaluation for an underlying malignancy are important, and both diseases have shown a strong association with myelogenous leukemia. These diagnoses are of exclusion, and infectious causes of blisters and ulcerations should be excluded with a tissue culture.[28,29]

Treatment/further work-up
Systemic corticosteroids can be initiated when infection has been excluded. These disorders may require a longer course of therapy with corticosteroids or steroid-sparing agents such as dapsone, potassium iodide, and colchicine. Work-up to determine an underlying cause is critical.[28,29]

Small Vessel Vasculitis

Background
Small vessel vasculitis may occasionally present with blisters, and can have multiple causes, including medications and autoimmune, infections, paraneoplastic, and idiopathic causes.[14] Because the pathogenesis involves immune complex deposition on small vessel endothelium, the subsequent vascular destruction and erythrocyte extravasation lead to focal skin necrosis, with hemorrhagic blistering as a consequence.

History
Patients can present with a variety of symptoms based on cause. Pruritus can be associated with drug-induced vasculitis, and systemic symptoms can occur with connective tissue diseases, infections, and with paraneoplastic causes.[14]

Physical examination
Palpable purpura can precede hemorrhagic vesicles typically on the lower extremities. These lesions then progress to ulceration.[14]

Diagnostic study/biopsy
Biopsy shows small vessel leukocytoclastic vasculitis.[14] Further testing is based on suspicion for underlying causes.

Treatment
If the cause is idiopathic and removal of a possible underlying cause fails to resolve the vasculitis, systemic corticosteroids are the mainstay of treatment. Dapsone, colchicine, and immunosuppressive medications can be considered as steroid-sparing therapy.[14]

INFECTIOUS VESICULOBULLOUS DERMATOSES

Several bacterial, viral, and fungal infections can present with vesicles and bullae (**Table 4**).[3,11,12,30–32] Herpes infections usually present as localized or dermatomal

Table 4
Infectious bullous diseases

Form of Infection	Clinical Characteristics	Diagnosis and Management
HSV	• HSV-1 and HSV-2 (most prevalent serotypes) • Predominantly orolabial (vermillion border) and genital. Occasionally, also seen on buttocks, finger (herpetic whitlow), face, and other sites of contact (herpes gladiatorum) • Vesicles and erosions in a cluster preceded by burning and pain • Primary infection: occurs within a week after exposure. Usually accompanied by symptoms of fatigue, lymphadenopathy, and occasional fevers. Takes 2–6 wk to resolve • Recurrent HSV infections: spontaneous or secondary to stress, UV light, or immunosuppression. Usually takes 7–10 d to resolve and are mild compared with primary HSV • Immunocompromised: tend to have disseminated vesicles and are at risk for systemic involvement. Cutaneous findings: atypical with persistent enlarging ulcerations, as well as verrucous lesions oddly distributed in some cases on the tongue, esophagus, and gastrointestinal mucosa • Disseminated form: also seen in patients with extensive skin barrier breakdown such as eczema	• Diagnostic tests: Tzanck smear, DFA, viral culture, serology and VZV PCR. Biopsy shows viral cytopathologic changes • Recurrent genital herpes: oral acyclovir (800 mg PO bid × 5d), valacyclovir(1 g PO qd × 5 d), and famciclovir(1 g PO bid × 1 d) can be used in immunocompetent hosts. A protracted course is used in the setting of orolabial herpes flare • Immunocompromised: disseminated HSV requires IV acyclovir at 10 mg/kg every 8 h in most cases or 1 g PO bid valacyclovir until all cutaneous lesions have resolved. Foscarnet may be used in resistant cases • >6 episodes a year: chronic suppressive therapy with acyclovir (400–800 mg PO bid to tid), or valacyclovir (500 mg qd to 1 g qd PO bid), or famciclovir (250 mg PO bid) is recommended

(continued on next page)

Table 4
(continued)

Form of Infection	Clinical Characteristics	Diagnosis and Management
VZV	• Primary varicella infection (chicken pox): prodromal systemic symptoms such as fevers and malaise with subsequent erythematous papulopustular eruption that then progress to vesicles on an erythematous base predominantly on the trunk with significant pruritus. Lesions at a given time can be at any stage of development. The lesions crust over within 10 d. Adults may have systemic complications such as pneumonia • Herpes zoster: prodromal burning pain or itching with subsequent development of clustered vesicles on an erythematous base in a dermatomal distribution usually on the trunk. They seldom cross the midline. Occasionally they can progress to bullae. Elderly or immunocompromised patients may develop postherpetic neuralgia with burning pain in the affected distribution. Pneumonitis and hepatitis occasionally develop • Immunocompromised: can have a more disseminated presentation with more than 20 vesicles outside of the dermatome along with occasional internal organ involvement	• Diagnostic tests: Tzanck smear, DFA, viral culture, serology, and VZV PCR • Biopsy shows viral cytopathologic changes • Varicella zoster immunoglobulin within 4 d of exposure can be considered in immunocompromised and pregnant women along with neonates without previous immunity • Primary varicella infection: acyclovir (20 mg/kg PO qid × ×5 d) or Valacyclovir (20 mg/kg PO tid × 5 d) is the treatment of choice • Reactivation: valacyclovir 1 g tid × 7 d with optimal results if treatment is initiated within 3 d of presentation. Oral acyclovir and famciclovir can also be used • Immunocompromised: IV acyclovir10 mg/kg every 8 h for 7-10 days or until lesions healed in some cases • In patients with postherpetic neuralgia, treatment with gabapentin or tricyclic antidepressants should be considered. Topical options include lidocaine creams, and 8% capsaicin patch • VZV live viral vaccine is effective in children • VZV vaccine is recommended for patients older than 60 y to prevent development of zoster and decrease the incidence of postherpetic neuralgia
Bullous impetigo	• Results from *Staphylococcus aureus*–derived local exfoliative toxin, which binds to a desmosomal protein leading to a blister formation. It is the same exfoliative toxin that mediates staphylococcal skin syndrome • It is usually seen in newborns and presents as small vesicles that progress to flaccid blisters that easily rupture leaving a collaret of scale predominantly on the trunk, axillae, face, buttock, and extremities • This is more localized, in contrast with staphylococcal scalded skin syndrome(also seen in children), which presents with diffuse erythema, flaccid bulla with positive Nikolsky sign, positive Asboe-Hansen sign, peeling, and erosions with accentuation in the intertriginous folds and perioral furrowing • Adult patients SSSS are typically more ill and complain of severe generalized skin tenderness. They have a prodrome of conjunctivitis, pharyngitis, and fever	• Culture: blister fluid usually grows S aureus. Biopsy shows acantholysis in the granular layer of the skin • Treatment: it usually resolves on its own by 6 wk. Topical antibiotic creams such as mupirocin, retapamulin, or fusidic acid can be used as first line and IV ceftriaxone can be used for complicated cases such as concomitant cellulitis or in patients with poor immunity • In adults, the mortality for SSSS is high and is seen most commonly in immunosuppressed individuals with HIV and renal failure. • Isolation of exotoxin A and B may be difficult • Biopsy usually shows intraepidermal split. Blood cultures are positive in adults more often than in children • Toxic shock syndrome and TEN are on the differential • Pneumonia is the most frequent complication

Bullous cellulitis	• Severe cases of cellulitis can actually present with vesicles and bullae overlying the erythematous, swollen, very painful, and poorly defined areas of involvement (usually unilateral) • Systemic symptoms of fatigue and fever typically precede the skin presentation • Most common causes: S aureus and GAS • Immunocompromised: mixed flora • Long-term monitoring: renal function for acute glomerulonephritis in the setting of GAS cellulitis	• Mostly a clinical diagnosis • Differential diagnosis: deep venous thrombosis, superficial thrombophlebitis, and stasis dermatitis • Treatment: oral antibiotics in most cases. IV antibiotics (usually reserved for patients with complicated cellulitis) • Recurrent cellulitis: most common in patients with stasis dermatitis. These patients should also be evaluated for interdigital macerations and tinea pedis
V vulnificus	• Vibrio skin infection usually presents with violaceous purpuric macules that progress to hemorrhagic bullae and vesicles that can ulcerate • Severe complications: sepsis and necrotizing fasciitis • It is mostly seen in men more than 40 y of age with exposure of open wounds to warm coastal seawater and/or raw seafood (shellfish) • Risk factors: diabetes, hemochromatosis, cirrhosis, antacid use, renal disease, as well as immunosuppression	• Wound culture: confirms the diagnosis • Pseudomonas infection should be considered on the differential diagnosis • Treatment: combination of doxycycline and IV ceftriaxone. Other alternatives are cefotaxime or ciprofloxacin • Given high mortality from sepsis, prompt empiric treatment within 24 h is indicated • Surgical debridement and occasionally amputation may be needed in severe cases with rapidly expanding bullae
Bullous tinea	• Inflammatory variant of tinea pedis can present with vesicles and bullae, especially on the medial foot • Severe cases may present with a concomitant id reaction/dermatophytid response with poorly demarcated symmetric eczematous patches in distant sites such as the face and extremities	• Fungal culture: Trichophyton mentagrophytes (most common) • Treatment: topical antifungal such as econazole or terbinafine cream is usually sufficient. In severe cases especially with id reaction and/or onychomycosis, consider oral antifungals (fluconazole and terbinafine). We recommend avoidance of oral ketoconazole because of inherent greater hepatic risks

Abbreviations: bid, twice a day; d, days; DFA, direct fluorescent antibody; GAS, group A Streptococcus; h, hours; HSV, herpes simplex virus; IV, intravenous; Kg, kilogram; mg, milligram; PO, orally; qd, every day; qid; S aureus, staphylococcus aureus; SSSS, staphylococcal scalded skin syndrome; TEN, toxic epidermal necrolysis; 4 times a day; tid, 3 times a day; UV, ultraviolet; VZV, varicella zoster virus; wk, weeks; y, years.

vesicles, but are occasionally disseminated or form bullae in immunocompromised hosts.[3] Tinea pedis (especially zoophilic species such as *Trichophyton mentagrophytes*) can present as vesicles and bullae on the bilateral feet, which can often be confused with ACD from footwear.[32] *Staphylococcus aureus* produces exotoxins against desmoglein-1 that result in bullous impetigo when localized and SSSS when systemic.[31] *V vulnificus* presents acutely with hemorrhagic blisters and sepsis.[11] Treatment and management depend on the type of infection and extent of involvement. Immunocompromised hosts tend to have more extensive involvement and generally require more aggressive therapy.[3]

BULLOUS DRUG ERUPTIONS

This entity consists of different vesiculobullous eruptions seen in the setting of medications, as detailed in **Table 3**.[14,33] Note that although some drug-induced reactions result in cytotoxic or cytokine-induced necrosis of keratinocytes (eg, fixed drug eruption or Stevens-Johnson syndrome [SJS]/TEN), others can result in drug-induced autoantibody-mediated bullous diseases, such as vancomycin-induced linear IgA bullous dermatosis. Management includes discontinuation of the medication along with management of symptoms. Some acute severe reactions, such as SJS/TEN, require an urgent multidisciplinary approach along with ophthalmology and a burn team.[12]

ACKNOWLEDGMENT

The authors would like to thank Samuel Kwak for his help with the images.

REFERENCES

1. Fine J-D, Mellerio JE. Epidermolysis Bullosa. In: Bolognia JL, Jorizzo JL, Schaffer JV, editors. Dermatology. 3rd edition. London: Saunders; 2012. p. 501–13.
2. Kneisel A, Hertl M. Autoimmune bullous skin diseases. Part 1: clinical manifestations. J Dtsch Dermatol Ges 2011;9(10):844–56 [quiz: 857].
3. Mendoza N, Madkan V, Sra K, et al. Human Herpes Viruses. In: Bolognia JL, Jorizzo JL, Schaffer JV, editors. Dermatology. 3rd edition. London: Saunders; 2012. p. 1321–43.
4. Johnston GA. Treatment of bullous impetigo and the staphylococcal scalded skin syndrome in infants. Expert Rev Anti Infect Ther 2004;2(3):439–46.
5. Contestable JJ, Edhegard KD, Meyerle JH. Bullous systemic lupus erythematosus: a review and update to diagnosis and treatment. Am J Clin Dermatol 2014;15(6):517–24.
6. Schulenburg-Brand D, Katugampola R, Anstey AV, et al. The cutaneous porphyrias. Dermatol Clin 2014;32(3):369–84, ix.
7. Vereecken P, Tas S, Verraes S, et al. Phototoxic contact phytodermatitis: clinical and biological aspects. Rev Médicale Brux 1998;19(3):131–4 [in French].
8. Almahameed A, Pinto DS. Pernio (chilblains). Curr Treat Options Cardiovasc Med 2008;10(2):128–35.
9. Mota ANC de M, Nery NS, Barcaui CB. Case for diagnosis: bullosis diabeticorum. An Bras Dermatol 2013;88(4):652–4.
10. Frank J, Poblete-Gutierrez P. Porphyria. In: Bolognia JL, Jorizzo JL, Schaffer JV, editors. Dermatology. 3rd edition. London: Saunders; 2012. p. 717–27.

11. Hsiao C-T, Lin L-J, Shiao C-J, et al. Hemorrhagic bullae are not only skin deep. Am J Emerg Med 2008;26(3):316–9.
12. Levitt J, Markoff B. Vesiculobullous skin disease. Hosp Med Clin 2014;3(4): 582–96.
13. Hull CM, Zone JJ. Dermatitis Herpetiformis and Linear IgA Bullous Dermatosis. In: Bolognia JL, Jorizzo JL, Schaffer JV, editors. Dermatology. 3rd edition. London: Saunders; 2012. p. 491–500.
14. Mascaro Jr. J. Other Vesiculobullous diseases. In: Bolognia JL, Jorizzo JL, Schaffer JV, editors. Dermatology. 3rd edition. London: Saunders; 2012. p. 515–22.
15. Amagai M. Pemphigus. In: Bolognia JL, Jorizzo JL, Schaffer JV, editors. Dermatology. 3rd edition. London: Saunders; 2012. p. 461–74.
16. Bernard P, Borradoria L. Pemphigoid Group. In: Bolognia JL, Jorizzo JL, Schaffer JV, editors. Dermatology. 3rd edition. London: Saunders; 2012. p. 475–90.
17. Nosbaum A, Vocanson M, Rozieres A, et al. Allergic and irritant contact dermatitis. Eur J Dermatol 2009;19(4):325–32.
18. Usatine RP, Riojas M. Diagnosis and management of contact dermatitis. Am Fam Physician 2010;82(3):249–55.
19. Cohen D, Souza AD. Irritant Contact dermatitis. In: Bolognia JL, Jorizzo JL, Schaffer JV, editors. Dermatology. 3rd edition. London: Saunders; 2012. p. 249–59.
20. Reider N, Fritsch PO. Other Eczematous Eruptions. In: Bolognia JL, Jorizzo JL, Schaffer JV, editors. Dermatology. 3rd edition. London: Saunders; 2012. p. 219–31.
21. McGovern TW. Dermatoses due to plants. In: Bolognia JL, Jorizzo JL, Schaffer JV, editors. Dermatology. 3rd edition. London: Saunders; 2012. p. 279–81.
22. Bottoni U, Mauro FR, Cozzani E, et al. Bullous lesions in chronic lymphocytic leukaemia: pemphigoid or insect bites? Acta Derm Venereol 2006;86(1):74–6.
23. Baum S, Sakka N, Artsi O, et al. Diagnosis and classification of autoimmune blistering diseases. Autoimmun Rev 2014;13(4–5):482–9.
24. Otten JV, Hashimoto T, Hertl M, et al. Molecular diagnosis in autoimmune skin blistering conditions. Curr Mol Med 2014;14(1):69–95.
25. Huilaja L, Mäkikallio K, Tasanen K. Gestational pemphigoid. Orphanet J Rare Dis 2014;9:136.
26. Cole MB, Smith ML. Environment and Sports-Related Skin Diseases. In: Bolognia JL, Jorizzo JL, Schaffer JV, editors. Dermatology. 3rd edition. London: Saunders; 2012. p. 1492–4.
27. Chacon AH, Farooq U, Choudhary S, et al. Coma blisters in two postoperative patients. Am J Dermatopathol 2013;35(3):381–4.
28. Sakiyama M, Kobayashi T, Nagata Y, et al. Bullous pyoderma gangrenosum: A case report and review of the published work. J Dermatol 2012;39(12):1010–5.
29. Voelter-Mahlknecht S, Bauer J, Metzler G, et al. Bullous variant of Sweet's syndrome. Int J Dermatol 2005;44(11):946–7.
30. Millett CR, Halpern AV, Reboli AC, et al. Bacterial diseases. In: Bolognia JL, Jorizzo JL, Schaffer JV, editors. Dermatology. 3rd edition. London: Saunders; 2012. p. 1187–220.
31. Patel GK, Finlay AY. Staphylococcal scalded skin syndrome: diagnosis and management. Am J Clin Dermatol 2003;4(3):165–75.
32. El-Segini Y, Schill W-B, Weyers W. Case Report. Bullous tinea pedis in an elderly man. Mycoses 2002;45(9–10):428–30.
33. Revuz J, Laurence V-A. Drug Reactions. In: Bolognia JL, Jorizzo JL, Schaffer JV, editors. Dermatology. 3rd edition. London: Saunders; 2012. p. 335–56.

Neurotoxins and Dermal Fillers: Choosing the Right Product

Risha Bellomo, MPAS, PA-C*, Lewis Kevin Harrington, ARNP, FNP-C

KEYWORDS

- Dermal fillers • Neurotoxins • Aesthetic medicine • Panfacial rejuvenation

KEY POINTS

- An understanding is needed of the current market for neurotoxin and dermal filler choices and how to differentiate products from one another.
- Physician assistants must understand the mechanism of action, proper reconstitution, unit dosing, and treatment areas of neurotoxins.
- There is a proper way to the panfacial approach to the aesthetic patient.
- There must be an understanding of the difference in dermal fillers, correct tissue placement, injection techniques, and how complications are avoided.

For more than 20 years physicians have been using Botulinum neurotoxin type A (BoNT-A) for medical and cosmetic uses. In 2008 there were 2.5 million procedures performed with BoNT-A and in 2014 that number increased to 3,588,218 as surveyed by the American Society for Aesthetic Plastic Surgery.[1] The current trend for cosmetic procedures is a nonsurgical approach, encompassing 83% of all cosmetic procedures.[2] BoNT-A is the most common and popular cosmetic procedure in women older than age 35 and men have been joining in to reap the benefits of such a safe and efficacious product.[2] Over the last 5 years there has been a significant increase in nonsurgical procedures for men with BoNT-A, up 84% and hyaluronic acid (HA) dermal fillers up 94%.[1]

Neurotoxins are only part of the equation to achieve panfacial aesthetic enhancement. With the wide array of choices on the market it can be difficult for a provider to know which dermal filler to choose. From treating lips and perioral lines to lifting and volumizing the mid-face the choices range from HAs, calcium hydroxyapatite (Radiesse), Artefill, and poly-L-lactic acid (Sculptra).

Disclosure Statement: R. Bellomo has no disclosures and K. Harrington is a trainer for Allergan.
Allele Medical, 2504 S. Alafaya Trail, Ste. 310, Orlando, FL 32828, USA
* Corresponding author.
E-mail address: RISHAPAC@YAHOO.COM

Physician Assist Clin 1 (2016) 333–345
http://dx.doi.org/10.1016/j.cpha.2015.12.008
2405-7991/16/$ – see front matter © 2016 Elsevier Inc. All rights reserved.

THE FIRST STEP: ASSESSING THE COSMETIC PATIENT

Patients seeking aesthetic enhancement are looking to maximize, recapture, or maintain their youthful appearance; maintain and restore a healthy appearance; and look as good as they feel. To achieve successful and desired outcomes the first steps are understanding the patient's needs, setting realistic expectations, and taking a panfacial approach to the evaluation. This panfacial approach includes identifying the aesthetic deficits of the entire face, but assessment of the neck, décolletage, and the dorsum of the hands is just as important.

It is recommended to start the evaluation by taking photographs and using those photographs as a tool for the initial consultation. Photographs should include frontal repose, frontal animated, and bilateral 45° and 90° positions. This allows the patient to visualize all panfacial views and gives the provider a more efficient tool to set expectations and explain the use of products for best outcomes. Identifying areas of concern initiates a conversation about treatment options and gives the clinician opportunity to develop an individualized annual cosmetic plan for the patient. For example, a patient presents to your office with dynamic and static rhytids of the glabellar complex, horizontal forehead lines, periorbital rhytids, and bunny lines. This patient is also concerned about deepening nasolabial folds, and thinning of the lips and perioral lip lines. On examination, it is also noted that the left cheek is becoming flat and not as prominent as the right. The next step is to discuss the treatment options for each area. Neurotoxins (Botox, Dysport, and Xeomin) are all adequate options for the glabellar, forehead, and periorbital lines, and for the treatment of bunny lines (nasalis). There are several dermal fillers to choose for mid-face volumizing, including Radiesse, Voluma, Sculptra, and Restylane Lyft. Restylane, Juvederm Ultra Plus, Juvederm Ultra, Restylane Lyft, ArteFill, and Radiesse are options for the nasolabial folds depending on severity of wrinkle assessment. Restylane Silk or Belotero are excellent choices for perioral rhytids and accentuating the vermillion border of the lips. Restylane and Juvederm Ultra are commonly used in the vermillion or the wet to dry area of the lips to create lip fullness.

There are several neurotoxins and dermal fillers to choose from. So how does one choose the correct product for patients? Having an understanding of product composition, longevity, mechanism of action, safety, shelf life and product cost is crucial in selecting the best products to meet your patient needs.

HISTORY OF THE FIRST BOTULINUM NEUROTOXIN TYPE A: BOTOX COSMETIC (onobotulinumtoxinA)

Botulinum toxin dates back to 1895 when the bacteria *Clostridium botulinum* was first identified. In the 1940s, Dr Edward J. Schantz and colleagues were able to purify the botulinum toxin. But it was not until the 1970s when the physician Allan Scott (considered the grandfather of BoNT-A) started to use BoNT-A for the medical treatment of strabismus and involuntary muscle spasms. In 1987, Jean Carruthers, an ophthalmologist, and her husband Alastair Carruthers, a dermatologist, started to experiment with BoNT-A in cosmetic dermatology. They found while using botulinum toxin for medical ophthalmic uses that the rhytids of the lateral orbicularis oculi started to diminish.[3] In 1989, BoNT-A was approved by the Food and Drug Administration (FDA) for the treatment of strabismus and blepharospasm and in 2000 it was approved for cervical dystonia. The initial name given to BoNT-A was Ocululinum; it was changed to Botox in 1991 when Allergan acquired the rights to the product. In the early 1990s, the Carruthers did the first studies of BoNT-A and they published their first paper on the potential of onabotulinumA in the field of cosmetic dermatology.[2] Finally in

April 2002, Botox was FDA approved for the treatment of moderate to severe glabellar lines in adult patients 65 years of age and younger. Two years later Botox was approved for severe primary axillary hyperhidrosis.[4,5] As of 2015, Botox is approved for the treatment of upper limb spasticity, overactive bladder, urinary incontinence, migraine headaches, cervical dystonia, severe primary axillary hyperhidrosis, blepharospasm, strabismus, moderate to severe frown lines of the glabellar complex, and crow's feet.[4]

Mechanism of Action of Botulinum Neurotoxin Type A

The clostridial neurotoxin is a polypeptide chain and has seven distinct sertotypes A through G, with types A and B being commercially available. The mechanism of action of BoNT-A is as follows (**Fig. 1**):

- A purified protein (contains no live bacteria)
- Targets localized selective muscles blocking neuromuscular transmission
- Binds to acceptor sites on presynaptic motor nerve terminals
- Proteases cleave the SNAP 25 protein, associated with the snare complex inhibiting the release of acetylcholine
- This produces a partial chemical denervation resulting in reduction of muscle activity
- This in turn relaxes the fine lines and wrinkles associated with the underlying muscle movement

Since April 2002, cosmetic dermatologists and plastic surgeons in the United States only had one FDA approved neurotoxin to choose from. But as of 2015 the FDA has approved abobotulinumtoxinA (Dysport) and incobotulinumtoxinA (Xeomin) for the temporary treatment of moderate to severe glabellar rhytids in patients younger than age 65 years.

AbobotulinumtoxinA was first used in Europe and was FDA approved in April 2009 in the United States. IncobotulinumtoxinA was FDA approved in 2010 for the treatment

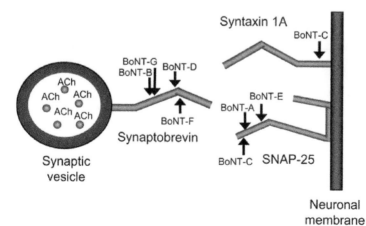

Fig. 1. Molecular targets of clostridial neurotoxins in presynaptic cell. BoNT/A-G, botulinum toxin A-G; TeNT, tetanus toxin. (*From* Barr JR, Moura H, Boyer AE, et al. Botulinum neurotoxin detection and differentiation by mass spectrometry. Emerg Infect Dis 2005;11(10):1578–83.)

of moderate to severe glabellar rhytids and was available to health care providers in 2012. All three neurotoxins have similar side effect and adverse reaction profiles. They vary in their molecular composition, reconstitution, and unit dosing (**Boxes 1–3, Table 1**).

When comparing Botox with Dysport one appreciates some clinical and technical differences. Note there have been no direct head-to-head studies between the two products. Starting with onset of effect, Dysport has shown to have a 50% response rate within 2 days, 70% to 80% by Days 3 and 4, and 90% response rate by Day 7. In clinical practice Botox onset of effect seems to take longer than Dysport, but the package insert does state the onset of action is 1 to 2 days. On initial visit at Day 7 of the clinical trials with Botox it was found the responder rate was 82.5% subject assessment.[4] Durations of both products seem to be similar, lasting on average 117 days.[2] Although there is some literature that states Dysport lasts longer than Botox this has yet to be proved. The two biggest differences between the products is the difference in unit dosing and diffusion ratios or field of effect (FOE). Dose equivalence between Botox and Dysport is the major question many clinicians have been wanting answered since Dysport was approved by the FDA.

Several studies have been conducted to determine dose equivalences between these two products but the question has yet to be answered scientifically. For example, one study concluded that Botox and Dysport had a similar FOE when measuring anhidrosis and muscle activity at a dose equivalence of 1.0 to 2.0 with significantly greater fields of anhidrotic effect at a dose equivalence of 1.0 to 2.5.[6] A different study published in 2013 measured the FOE by observing anhidrotic effects, evoked compound muscle action potentials, and wrinkle assessment as measured by a four-point validated wrinkle assessment scale.[7] Nineteen participants were injected with 2 U of onabotulinumtoxinA in one side of the forehead and 2 U of abobotulinumtoxinA on the other side. The results reported were significantly larger FOE with onabotulinumbtoxinA than for abobotulinumtoxinA with no significant differences between the two products for evoked compound muscle action potentials or wrinkle assessment score at Day 28. The authors concluded that "Although many studies state that diffusion is product dependent and abobotulinumtoxinA diffuses more

---

Box 1
Contraindications and precautions for Botox and Xeomin

Contraindications

The only contraindications for Botox and Xeomin are known hypersensitivities to any ingredient and infection at the injection sites

For Dysport, the addition of allergies to cow's milk protein

Precautions

Pregnancy and nursing

Neurologic conditions, such as myasthenia gravis

Lambert-Eaton syndrome, amyotrophic lateral sclerosis (Lou Gehrig disease)

Some autoimmune conditions

Data from Botox cosmetic (botulinum toxin type A) purified neurotoxin complex [package insert]. Irvine, CA: Allergan, Inc; and Dysport [package insert]. Scottsdale, AZ: Medicis, Inc.

Box 2
Theoretic drug interactions

Aminoglycoside antibiotics

Cyclosporine

Calcium channel blockers

Cholinesterase inhibitors

Data from Botox cosmetic (botunlinum toxin type A) purified neurotoxin complex [package insert]. Irvine, CA) Allergan, Inc; and Dysport [package insert]. Scottsdale, AZ: Medicis, Inc.

---

than onabotulinumtoxinA, findings from the present study confirm that diffusion is dose dependent and the more potent dose tested diffuses more."[7]

As is evident by the conflicting results of the two previously mentioned studies, dose equivalence has not been established. This supports the statement that the units of neurotoxins are not interchangeable and it seems that the strength of dosing is the major contributor to product diffusion.

As stated in the package insert, under Warnings and Precautions, there is a "lack of interchangeability between Botulinum Toxin Products."[4] All neurotoxins are dosed in units that measure the toxin activity. Each manufacturer has its own unique formulation, therefore units to measure the activity of one product cannot be used to measure the activity of another.[4,8,9] **Table 2** provides information regarding dilutions.

The neurotoxin core is 150 kDa in its pure form and is not variable. Each neurotoxin has its own pharmacokinetics, properties, and characteristics. It is important to have a clear understanding of the differences among the three commercially available neurotoxins.

Xeomin is considered the pure neurotoxin, which is different compared with the other neurotoxins approved by the FDA. During the manufacturing process the accessory proteins are removed leaving only the therapeutic core. This feature, although not scientifically proven, is thought to potentially decrease the immunologic resistance because of neutralizing antibodies. It is also thought to decrease the chance of an

---

Box 3
Side effects/adverse reactions

Headache

Respiratory infections

Eyelid ptosis

Brow ptosis

Bruising

Swelling

Numbness/tingling

Nausea

Flulike symptoms

Diplopia

Data from Botox cosmetic (botunlinum toxin type A) purified neurotoxin complex [package insert]. Irvine, CA: Allergan, Inc; and Dysport [package insert]. Scottsdale, AZ: Medicis, Inc.

Table 1
Aesthetic uses of neurotoxins and muscles treated

Aesthetic Uses of Neurotoxins	Muscles Treated
Glabellar rhytids (only on-label use)	Procerus, corrugators
Horizontal forehead lines	Frontalis
Crow's feet	Orbicularis oculi
Bunny lines	Nasalis
Downturned mouth	Depressor anguli oris
Mental crease/dimpling chin	Mentalis
Gummy smile	Levator labi superioris alaeque nasi
Nasal tip elevation	Depressor septi
Vertical lip lines	Orbicularis oris
Platysmal bands	Platysma
Facial narrowing from large masseters	Masseters

allergic reaction to the neurotoxin. The rate of immunologic resistance has been documented to be as high as 10% and as low as 3%.[10] Xeomin, although new in the United States, was first introduced in Germany in 2005 for the treatment of blepharospasm and cervical dystonia. Xeomin is the first neurotoxin that can remain at room temperature before reconstitution, but should be refrigerated after reconstitution. The manufacturer states that Xeomin is stable for 3 years at room temperature and newer studies have shown stability at 4 years.[10] Xeomin is the most cost-effective neurotoxin for health care providers to purchase, averaging $453 for a 100-U vial (**Table 3**).

When considering individualized treatment with neurotoxins the following should be considered: variations in patient's aesthetic goals; variables that would impact selected dosing as it relates to gender, muscle mass, action, and wrinkle pattern; areas to be treated; anatomic variation, symmetry, asymmetry; and patient's aesthetic preference. Does the patient want a "natural look" or a "done look"? Because there is no standardized dosing for neurotoxins it is important to choose a starting point and develop the appropriate dose for each patient. Remember, men typically need larger dosing than women related to their increased muscle mass. The guidelines listed in **Table 4** are a starting point for dosing, but these are only guidelines and each patient should be evaluated individually to achieve excellent cosmetic outcomes.

When treating platysmal bands it is important to be conservative and only experienced injectors should treat this area. Possible adverse reactions include difficulty swallowing, neck weakness, asymmetric smiling, and dry mouth.

Table 2
Dilutions

Saline Diluent Volume, mL	Botox, U/0.1 mL	Xeomin, U/0.1 mL	Dysport, U/0.1 mL
1.0	10	10	30
1.5	6.7	6.7	20
2.0	5.0	5.0	15
2.5	4.0	4.0	12
3.0	3.3	3.3	10

Data from Kane MAC. Advances in cosmetic therapy: a focus on BoNT-A. Medicis. Accessed July 2009.

Table 3
Technical variables

Botox	Dysport	Xeomin
Allergan, Inc	Galderma	Merz Pharmaceuticals
OnaotulinumA	AbobotulinumA	IncobotulinumA
50-, 100-U Vial	500-U vial	50-, 100-U Vial
900 kDa	300–900 kDa	150 kD
Human serum albumin	Human serum albumin	Human serum albumin
NaCl	Lactose	Sucrose
Complexing proteins	Complexing proteins	No complexing proteins
Shelf Life		
36 mo	6 mo	36–48 mo
Storage		
2° to 8°	2° to 8°	Room temperature
Biologic activity in relation to Botox		
1	1/3	1

Adapted from Park J, Lee MS, Harrison AR. Profile of Xeomin (incobotulinumtoxinA) for the treatment of blepharospasm. Clin Ophthalmol 2011;5:725–32.

Neurotoxins in cosmetic dermatology continue to be the most common nonsurgical cosmetic procedure and with new neurotoxins coming to the market the choices clinicians are able to give patients and the cosmetic outcomes are limitless.

AESTHETIC ENHANCEMENT WITH A VARIETY OF DERMAL FILLERS

Aesthetic enhancement does not stop at neurotoxins. A conversation about dermal fillers is paramount to achieve superior cosmetic outcomes. Optimal aesthetic outcomes can be achieved with an increased knowledge of the products available and how to educate the patient as to which dermal filler is best suited for their individual cosmetic needs.

Hyaluronic Acid Dermal Fillers

Hyaluronic acid (HA) is a naturally occurring polysaccharide (a sugar) present in body tissues, such as in skin and cartilage. It is extremely hydrophilic, that is it attracts water, and this creates a swelling pressure that enables it to withstand compressive

Table 4
Guidelines for treatment-dose ranges

Area Treated	Units of Botox	Units of Dysport
Glabella	20–30	50–75
Forehead	10–20	25–50
Crow's feet	8–20 per side	16–60 per side
Bunny lines	5–10	10–30
Lateral brow lift	4–6	8–12
Downturned mouth	3–8 per side	6–20 per side
Mental crease/dimpling chin	3–10	6–25
Platysmal bands	10–15 per band	20–40 per band

forces making this an ideal substance for dermal fillers. The original FDA-approved HAs collected the HA from avian rooster combs, which in turn increased the risk of untoward immunologic effects. To decrease the risk of these side effects, and improve the safety profile of HA fillers, HA is now harvested from gram-positive bacteria.[11,12]

To decrease the degradation of the HA products postimplantation, manufacturers use a chemical cross-linking agent that binds the polysaccharide chains together.

Differentiating Hyaluronic Acid Dermal Fillers

Chemical cross-linking of HA gives the dermal filler a hydrogel matrix that is resistant to degradation and increases the longevity of the dermal filler once it is administered into the skin.[13] For this reason, HA dermal fillers show immediate results with little recovery time and a relatively long-lasting effect.[13] Each HA dermal filler differs in the amount of HA cross-linking. If a dermal filler has a higher degree of cross-linking the matrix is tightly packed, which leads to greater gel firmness. The greater the gel firmness the fewer changes in form caused by facial movements and increased longevity. Gel firmness can affect the extrusion force, which is how much force it takes to push the product through a needle of a certain gauge. Because of this, it is essential that the HA is sized correctly in the manufacturing process to lower the extrusion force and allow for a steady flow of product through a particular gauge needle. This process is called "gel calibration." Gel calibration is an essential component to allow ease of injection for a smooth and steady experience. It makes sense that the firmer a gel the larger the particle size and the larger the gauge of the needle.[13] Most FDA-approved HA fillers, except for Juvederm Voluma, are hydrophilic so one should slightly undercorrect the treatment area.

If treating lips or fine lines use a product that is soft, has less cross-linking, less gel calibration, and is more dispersible when placed in the lips or superficial dermis. By using a 30-gauge 0.5-inch needle the injector has better precision and a better overall result with a natural look.[13] Restylane Silk and Belotero have properties that make each of these products a good choice for lips, perioral rhytids, and tear troughs. Many HA products, including Restylane Silk and Belotero, use cross-linking agents, such as 1,4-butanediol diglycidal ether. The properties of HA dermal fillers and their proprietary manufacturing process allow for improved tissue integration.[14]

The injector has many choices for the treatment of nasolabial folds, so a thorough evaluation of the severity and depth of the nasolabial folds is imperative for optimal correction (**Fig. 2**, **Table 5**). FDA-approved and available HA dermal fillers are listed in **Table 6**.

Beyond Hyaluronic Acid Dermal Fillers: Radiesse, Sculptra, and Artefill

Radiesse

Radiesse is a semisolid, cohesive dermal filler composed of calcium hydroxyapatite microspheres suspended in a carboxymethylcellulose gel carrier intended for subdermal implantation. The microspheres range in size from 25 to 45 μm.[15] Radiesse is FDA approved for the treatment of moderate to severe wrinkles and folds, such as smile lines or nasolabial folds, and is approved for hand augmentation to correct volume loss in the dorsum of the hands.[16] Radiesse has been used to augment cheeks, temples, nasolabial folds, oral commissures, chin wrinkles, prejowl folds, and marionette lines making it an excellent choice for panfacial rejuvenation. Radiesse gives an immediate result and is an excellent product for lift capacity that can last for up to 1 year. It is recommended to use a 25-gauge 1-inch needle to decrease the extrusion force of Radiesse. Hand augmentation with Radiesse has become popular in recent months masking prominent veins and tendons and leaving the hands looking natural and

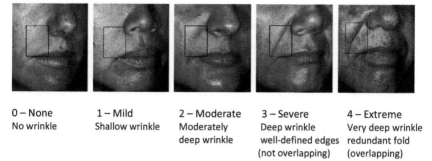

0 – None	1 – Mild	2 – Moderate	3 – Severe	4 – Extreme
No wrinkle	Shallow wrinkle	Moderately deep wrinkle	Deep wrinkle well-defined edges (not overlapping)	Very deep wrinkle redundant fold (overlapping)

Fig. 2. Nasolabial fold scale. (*From* Baumann LS, Shamban AT, Lupo MP, et al. Juvederm vs. Zyplast Nasolabial Fold Study Group. Dermatol Surg 2007;33(Suppl 2):S128–35; with permission.)

youthful. Radiesse is available in 0.8 mL and 1.5 mL.[16] Lip augmentation with Radiesse is not recommended because of an increased risk of nodules and granulomas.[15] Radiesse has no antidote and is not reversible.

Sculptra

Sculptra Aesthetic is an injectable poly-L-lactic acid bio-activator indicated for the use in patients with a healthy immune system as a single regimen for the correction of shallow to deep nasolabial fold contour deficiencies and other facial wrinkles in which deep dermal grid pattern or cross-hatch injection techniques is appropriate.[17] Sculptra was first FDA approved in 2004 for the treatment of lipoatrophy in patients with human immunodeficiency virus. In 2009, Sculptra received its FDA approval as a facial injectable for the correction of nasolabial folds and facial wrinkles. Poly-L-lactic acid is a synthetic material that works to replace lost collagen. It is safe and is absorbed naturally by the body. Sculptra is a biostimulator that stimulates fibroblasts to produce collagen, which thickens the dermis and gives the skin a healthy, youthful glow.[14] Patient education and setting initial expectations are crucial when choosing Sculptra for a patient's facial aesthetic needs. If the patient is expecting immediate results then this product is not for them. To achieve optimal results with Sculptra patients should receive three treatment sessions 4 to 6 weeks apart. I explain to my patients that they will start to see results as early as 2 to 3 months, but they will continue to see

Table 5
Dermal filler choices for nasolabial folds based on degree of wrinkle assessment and number of syringes to achieve full correction

Degree of Wrinkle Assessment	Type of Dermal Filler	# of Syringes
1. Mild	Restylane	1
	Juvederm Ultra	1
2. Moderate	Restylane	2
	Juvederm Ultra	2
3. Severe (may need to layer fillers; also treat mid-face)	Restylane Lyft	2
	Restylane	3
	Juvederm Ultra Plus	2
	Radiesse	2
4. Extreme (layer fillers; treat mid-face)	Radiesse	2–3
	Restylane Lyft	2
	Juvederm Ultra Plus	2

Table 6
FDA-approved and available HA dermal fillers

Manufacturer	Product Placement	FDA Approval
Allergan		
Juvederm Ultra Juvederm Ultra Plus	Mid to deep dermis	Correction of moderate to severe facial wrinkles and folds (eg, nasolabial folds)
Juvederm Voluma	Deep (subcutaneous and/or supraperiosteal)	Cheek augmentation to correct age-related volume deficit in the mid-face in adults older than 21 years of age
Merz		
Belotero Balance	Facial tissue	Smooth wrinkles and folds, around mouth and augmentation of lips
Galderma		
Restylane Silk	Dermis	Indicated for lip augmentation and dermal implantation for correction of perioral rhytids (wrinkles around the lips) in patients older than 21 years of age
Restylane	Mid to deep dermis	Correction of moderate to severe facial wrinkles/folds (eg, nasolabial folds) and for lip augmentation in those older than 21 years of age
Restylane Lyft (formerly marketed as Perlane-L)	Deep dermis to subcutaneous to supraperiosteal	Correction of moderate to severe facial wrinkles and folds (eg, nasolabial folds) Cheek augmentation and correction of age-related midface contour deficiencies in patients older than 21 years of age

Data from U.S. Food and Drug Administration. Soft tissue fillers approved by the center for devices and radiological health. Available at: http://www.fda.gov/MedicalDevices/ProductsandMedicalProcedures/CosmeticDevices/WrinkleFillers/ucm227749.htm.

improvement over a 6- to 9-month period. The results can last up to 18 to 24 months. Sculptra is the perfect choice for patients who have lost volume in the temporal region, mid-face, and lower face.

Bellafill

Bellafill was FDA approved in 2006 for the treatment and correction of nasolabial folds. Bellafill is composed of 80% purified bovine collagen sourced from the United States from a controlled and monitored herd and 20% polymethylmethacrylate microspheres. The microspheres are 30 to 50 μm in diameter and the product is highly purified to reduce immunogenicity.[14] The benefit of Bellafill is the longevity of the product making it a semipermanent dermal filler lasting up to 7 years. A skin test is required before treatment. The product is placed in the mid to deep dermis and is an excellent choice for the treatment of acne scarring. Unlike HAs that are able to be degraded by hyaluronidase, Bellafill has no reversible antidote. The ideal patient is an older patient looking for long-term outcomes who does not want to return for aesthetic treatments every 6 to 12 months.[14]

INJECTION TECHNIQUE IS CRITICAL FOR ADEQUATE CORRECTION

Injection techniques and depth placement of dermal fillers are key components to achieving full correction and successful outcomes. Proper injection technique also decreases risk of complications and adverse events. Patients should be seated upright in a 90 degree position to adequately visualize the rhytids and deficits.[18] The choice of injection technique depends on anatomic location, type of deficit, dermal filler used, and the individual patient.

Types of Injection Techniques

Serial puncture technique
Utilizes several needle punctures delivering a small amount of product in a precise manner. This does well in superficial lines, but one has to be cautious not to cause a Tyndall effect (bluish hue caused by the effect of light refraction through the skin layers hitting the injected product. This occurs when HA fillers are placed too superficially in the skin). This technique works well in shallow acne scarring, fine lines of the forehead and glabella, perioral rhytids, enhancement of the philtrum, and to add volume supraperiosteal. (note that when injecting supraperiosteal placement depth should be on top of bone).[18,19]

Linear threading injection technique
This uses a single linear thread of product that encompasses the entire length of the deficit. The advantages of this technique are a smooth, continuous line of product; fewer needle punctures; and less risk of injecting product into a vessel. This technique decreases bruising and swelling and is used best in the nasolabial folds and contouring the vermillion border.[18,19]

Fanning injection technique
This technique is used in combination with a liner, retrograde technique, but before withdrawing the needle from the skin the needle is adjusted gently in a different direction creating a fanning technique. This technique can be used in the nasolabial folds by directing medially and in the marionette lines and oral commissures. This technique also works well for mid-face contouring.[18,19]

Cross-hatching injection technique
This technique is similar to the linear technique, in which the direction of the needle is placed vertically and then horizontally. Cross-hatching uses linear threading to create several parallel linear threads and then perpendicular linear threads are laid across the initial threads. This technique provides the greatest lift and works best on larger area deficits, such as the cheeks or severe and extreme deficits of the nasolabial folds.[18,19]

Antegrade injection or push-ahead technique
This technique pushes product into the skin as one moves forward with the needle. This works well for downturned mouth, but caution should be used around areas of concern where vessels may become compromised (**Fig. 3**).[18,19]

Retrograde injection technique
This technique pushes product into the skin as one moves the needle backwards in a linear fashion. This works well for filling deficits of the nasolabial folds and tear troughs. (note when treating tear troughs, product must be placed supraperiosteal).

ADVERSE REACTIONS OF DERMAL FILLERS

There are several adverse reactions that can happen with the use of dermal fillers. The more common are temporary injection site redness, swelling, pain or tenderness, bruising, lumps, firmness, and itching and/or rash.[20] As with any implant or medication

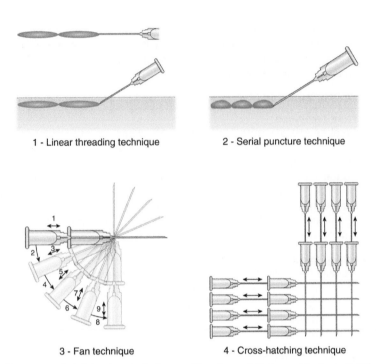

Fig. 3. Recommended injection techniques. (*Courtesy of* Pulmon Medical, Natal, South Africa. Available at: http://www.pulmonmedical.com.)

an allergic reaction is always possible. In addition, if one injects into or very close to a blood vessel it can cause ischemia or a necrotic event. It is good practice to aspirate before injecting the dermal filler into the tissue and to avoid highly vascular areas to prevent a vascular incident.

With the duration of dermal fillers increasing, clinicians must be educated about biofilm and different measures that can be taken to prevent infection of the implant. Hence, it is prudent to prepare the target injection site with a product that is bacteriocidal, such as chlorhexidine.

SUMMARY

With the invention of neurotoxins and dermal fillers clinicians can now effectively address facial changes associated with movement and the aging process without having surgery the only option. In just over a decade, facial rejuvenation has evolved into a combination of several different treatment modalities, such as skin care; skin cancer prevention; healthy eating; surgery; neurotoxins; dermal fillers; and skin rejuvenation technology, such as radiofrequency, light therapy, and lasers. Clinicians now understand to achieve panfacial rejuvenation and to meet the concerns and aesthetic needs of patients they must address the causes of facial changes associated with the aging process. Aesthetic medicine, and all of the product choices, can be overwhelming without continuing education. Product knowledge in conjunction with quality injection training allows clinicians to select the best treatment options to align with the patient's aesthetic goals to ensure superior patient outcomes.

REFERENCES

1. The American Society for Aesthetic Plastic Surgery reports Americans spent more than 12 billion in 2014. Procedures for men up 43% over five year period. Available at: http://www.surgery.org/media/news-releases/the-american-society-for-aesthetic-plastic-surgery-reports-americans-spent-more-than-12-billion-in-2014-pro. Accessed October 27, 2015.
2. Kane MA. Advances in cosmetic therapy: a focus on BoNT-A. Medicis. Available at: http://static1.1.sqspcdn.com/static/f/1062751/17362887/1332952456390/bonta-paper.pdf?token=HorjnLUxp4nzolgiba9ADJRT%2BGs%3D. Accessed July 2009.
3. Carruthers A, Carruthers J. Cosmetic uses for botulinum A exotoxin. Adv dermatol. In: Klein AS, editor. Tissue augmentation in clinical practice. Marcel Dekker, Inc; 1998. p. 207–36.
4. Botox cosmetic (botunlinum toxin type A) purified neurotoxin complex [package insert]. Irvine, (CA): Allergan, Inc.
5. Available at: https://common.wikimedia.org/wiki/File:Presynaptic_CNTs_targets.svg. Accessed July 2009.
6. Hexsel D, Brum C, do Prado DZ, et al. Field effect of two commercial preparations of botulinum toxin type A. J Am Acad Dermatol 2012;67(2):226–32.
7. Hexsel D, Hexsel C, Siega C. Fields of effects of 2 commercial preparations of botulinum toxin type A at equal labeled unit doses: a double-blind randomized trial. JAMA Dermatol 2013;149(12):1386–91.
8. Dysport [package insert]. Scottsdale, AZ: Medicis, Inc.
9. Hauser R, Wahba M, McClain TA. Botox (R) injections in plastic surgery. Available at: http://emedicine.medscape.com/article/1271380-overview. Accessed July 2009.
10. Park J, Lee MS, Harrison AR. Profile of Xeomin (incobotulinumtoxinA) for the treatment of blepharospasm. Clin Ophthalmol 2011;5:725–32. Accessed June 11, 2015.
11. Gold MH. Use of hyaluronic acid fillers for the treatment of the aging face. Clin Interv Aging 2007;2(3):369–76.
12. FDA. Products and medical procedures. Available at: http://www.fda.gov/MedicalDevices/ProductsandMedicalProcedures.
13. Segura S, Anthonioz L, Fuchez F, et al. A complete range of hyaluronic acid filler with distinctive physical properties specifically designed for optimal tissue adaptations. J Drugs Dermatol 2012;11(1 Suppl):s5–8.
14. Weinkle S, Gilbert E, Sadick N, et al. Expert profiles of filler for your practice. Practical Dermatology 2013;10(10):25–33.
15. Jacovella PF. Use of calcium hydroxylapatite (Radiesse)for facial augmentation. Clin Interv Aging 2008;3(1):161–74.
16. Radiesse [package insert]. Merz Aesthetics.
17. Sculptra aesthetic. Available at: http://www.sculptraaesthetic.com. Accessed June 11, 2015.
18. Grimes PE. Aesthetics and cosmetic surgery for darker skin types. Philadelphia: Lippincott Williams & Wilkins; 2008.
19. Carruthers A, Carruthers J. Procedures in cosmetic dermatology series: soft tissue augmentation. 3rd edition. Philadelphia: Saunders.
20. FDA. Medical devices. Soft tissue fillers (dermal fillers). Available at: http://www.fda.gov/medicaldevices/productsandmedicalprocedures/cosmeticdevices/wrinklefillers/default.htm.

Nail Findings
What Is a Provider to Do?

 CrossMark

Martha L. Sikes, MS, RPh, PA-C*, Philip E. Tobin, DHSc, PA-C

KEYWORDS

- Nail abnormalities • Beau lines • Mees lines • Terry nails • Onychomycosis
- Longitudinal melanonychia • Subungual hematoma • Nail matrix melanoma

KEY POINTS

- Nail disorders are common dermatologic conditions that warrant the provider to take a detailed history and perform a thorough examination of all 20 nails.
- Recognition of nonspecific and specific nail signs can direct providers to consider systemic disorders before patients presenting with systemic symptoms.
- Knowledge of normal nail anatomy is essential in determining the causes of nail disorders and their treatment.

INTRODUCTION

Nail disorders are a common presenting patient complaint and make up approximately 10% of all dermatologic conditions.[1] These disorders can occur throughout life but more often in the elderly population.[2] This occurrence is due in part to age-related nail changes, such as impaired peripheral circulation, long-term UV radiation exposure, trauma, infections, comorbid systemic diseases, polypharmacy, and the normal aging process.[2] As the nail ages, changes in mineral composition of the nail plate, keratinocyte size, growth rate, color, contour, texture, and thickness occur.[2] Knowledge of the normal nail anatomy, function of each nail unit structure, and growth rate provides clues to the provider to determine nail pathology. In some cases, fingernails function as an early warning system to alert the provider the patient may have a serious systemic illness before systemic manifestations become apparent.

Disclosure: None of the authors has any conflicts of interest associated with the work presented in this article.
Department of Physician Assistant Studies, Mercer University, 3001 Mercer University Drive, Atlanta, GA 30341, USA
* Corresponding author.
E-mail address: sikes_ml@mercer.edu

Physician Assist Clin 1 (2016) 347–361
http://dx.doi.org/10.1016/j.cpha.2015.12.009
2405-7991/16/$ – see front matter © 2016 Elsevier Inc. All rights reserved.
physicianassistant.theclinics.com

PARTS OF THE NAIL AND THEIR FUNCTION

Human fingernails have a rate of growth of around 0.1 mm per day, which translates into a 4- to 6-month time frame for the length of a fingernail to completely grow.[3] The nail unit itself is composed of the nail bed, matrix, proximal nail fold, and hyponychium; however, there are other structures associated with the nail (**Fig. 1**).[1]

- Nail plate: This part is the hard cutaneous portion made up of hard and soft keratin that provides protection to the nail unit. The normal pink appearance of the nail plate is due to the vascular layer of the nail bed.[1]
- Nail bed: This structure contains vascular capillaries and adheres to the nail plate. It begins where the lunula ends and extends to the hyponychium.[1] The ultimate function of the nail bed is to provide support to the nail plate.[4]
- Lunula: This part is the white, half-moon shaped area located at the proximal nail plate and represents the most distal portion of the nail matrix.[1] It ultimately determines the nail plate shape.[1]
- Nail folds: The proximal and lateral nail folds border the nail plate. Together they support and direct the growth process of the nail plate.[4] Around a quarter of the total surface area of the nail plate is located under the proximal nail fold.[1]
- Eponychium (cuticle): This structure consists of a portion of the proximal nail fold that seals the nail plate and helps provide protection against organisms that could affect the matrix.[1] Any alteration to the eponychium disrupts its barrier protection and can lead to inflammation and nail abnormalities.[1]
- Nail matrix: This area is where the nail is developed. It is the thick portion of the nail bed located under the proximal nail fold.[4]
- Hyponychium: This area is where the epidermis is located between the nail bed and the distal portion of the free edge of the nail plate. This structure functions in a similar manner as the eponychium in providing protection to the matrix.[1]

EVALUATION OF NAILS

A detailed history is an essential part in determining nail pathology.[4] During the nail examination, historical questions may need to be revisited in order to establish a proper timeline.

- How long has this condition been present?
- Which nails were affected first?
- Which nails are affected now?
- How has the presentation changed since you first noticed it?
- Has there been any previous trauma to the nails? This point is especially difficult for patients to remember; use normal nail growth times to determine when the event occurred in order to help trigger their memory.
- What is your occupation? Be sure to ask details about their daily workplace activities. Is there anything that may affect their nails such as exposure to chemicals, irritants, water, or even typing?
- What are your hobbies? Runners and other athletes are especially at risk of having nail deformities due to constant trauma to their nails.
- Do you have any nail habits, such as picking, biting, sucking, or cuticle manipulation? These habits may be apparent on general observation of patients.
- What is your normal nail care regimen? Be sure to ask about the use of nail polish, base/top coat, strengtheners, hardeners, conditioners, cuticle treatment, instruments used during nail care, manicures, and artificial or gel nails.

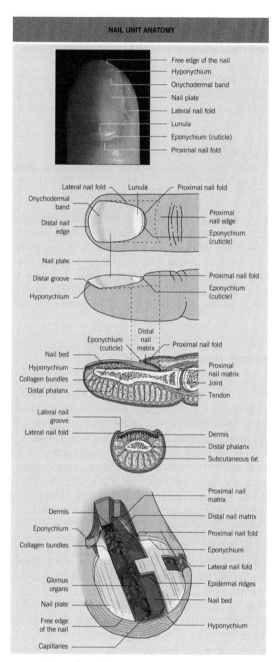

Fig. 1. Nail unit anatomy. (*From* de Berker D, Higgins CA, Jahoda C, et al. Biology of hair and nails. In: Bolognia JL, Jorizzo JL, Schaffer JV, editors. Dermatology. 3rd edition. Philadelphia: Elsevier/Saunders; 2012. p. 1075–92; with permission.)

- Do you have any other skin conditions, such as psoriasis, tinea pedis, tinea corporis, tinea cruris, lichen planus, or eczema?
- Do you have any other medical problems?
- What are you current medications?
- What medications have you taken in the past year? The year time frame for medication history is essential as medications are associated with certain nonspecific nail findings and patients may not be currently taking the medication that caused the nail disorder.
- Have you tried any self-treatment or medical treatments for your nail problem?
- Do you have any family history of nail problems?
- What type of diet do you typically eat? Certain nutritional deficiencies are associated with nail changes.

Physical examination
- It is vital that an inspection of all 20 nails, the perionychium (proximal and lateral nail folds), eponychium, hyponychium, lunula, and nail plate is performed.
- Note findings, such as pitting, onycholysis, nail color, nail plate consistency (brittle, peeling, thin, thick), and any horizontal or longitudinal lines.
- Systemic disorders may cause nail abnormalities, such as changes in shape, growth, or color. These findings may assist the provider in determining the diagnosis of specific disease states but are more commonly nonspecific reaction patterns.[3]

SELECTED COMMON NAIL FINDINGS
Beau Lines

A French physician in 1846 by the name of Joseph Honoré Simon Beau first described this nail alteration in a patient following a febrile illness.[5] Since that time, Beau lines have been reported to occur for a multitude of reasons and are one of the most common, but least specific, nail abnormalities.[4] The abnormality is thought to result from an interference with the blood supply and normal nail metabolism of the proximal nail matrix, although the true pathophysiology is poorly understood.[5] Patients typically present with a nonpainful transverse groove in the nail plate that progresses distally with nail growth. The nails will appear pink; it is most often bilateral, usually affects thumbnails and great toenails the most, and may be present in all 20 nails (**Fig. 2**).

Key history findings include:
- Medications used in the last 6–12 months such as chemotherapy drugs, oral retinoids, and a few other miscellaneous medications have been implicated in the development of these grooves.[5]
- Any recent illnesses, such as pneumonia, measles, mumps, scarlet fever, and other infections, have resulted in the Beau lines. High fever is also known to induce these lines.[5]
- Any injuries or trauma in the last six months may cause Beau lines to occur. These lines may present unilaterally if trauma of an upper limb (such as hand, finger, wrist, elbow, forearm), an inflammatory process, or neurologic event occurs.[5] As stated previously, providers may need to revisit this question after inspecting the nails and determining the timing of the initiating event.
- Any systemic disorders, including recent myocardial infarction, hyperthyroidism, diabetes mellitus, renal failure, gout, and severe epileptic seizure, have all been implicated in the development of Beau lines.[5]

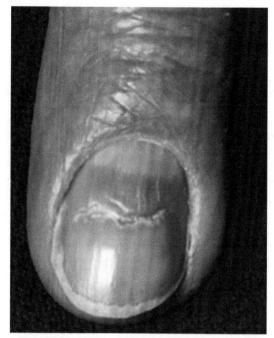

Fig. 2. Beau lines. (*From* James WD, Elston DM, Berger TG, et al. Andrews' diseases of the skin: clinical dermatology. 11th edition. London: Saunders/Elsevier; 2011. p. 741–82; with permission.)

- Cutaneous disease, such as eczema flares, pustular psoriasis, alopecia areata, or other inflammatory insults (ie, Steven Johnson syndrome or toxic epidermal necrolysis), may disrupt the function of the matrix.[5]
- Nutritional deficiencies, such as protein deficiency, pellagra, hypocalcemia, and zinc deficiency, have also been associated with this nail abnormality.[1,5]

Physical examination findings:

- Transverse furrows or grooves on the nail plate that may result in onychomadesis may be found.
- Providers should measure the space between the eponychium and groove to determine when arrest of the nail matrix occurred.
- In theory, the depth of the transverse groove may determine the severity of insult.[5]

The differential diagnosis for Beau lines typically includes trauma, Mees lines, and habit tick deformity. A detailed history will help narrow the cause. Routine laboratory workup is not necessary unless needed to determine any underlying systemic disorders.

Beau lines require no specific treatment, and the goal of therapy should be to identify and treat any underlying cause or remove the offending medication if possible. Providers should reassure patients this nail abnormality will resolve and include proper nail care counseling.

Mees Lines

Mees lines, also known as Aldrich-Mees lines, were first described by E. S. Reynolds in 1901, again in 1904 by C. J. Aldrich, and ultimately credited to R. A. Mees in 1919.

This physical finding was described by all 3 physicians in relation to arsenic poisoning. Mees lines are thought to occur from an abnormal keratinization of the nail plate following an injury to the nail matrix. Patients typically present with transverse, non-painful white bands on all fingernails (**Fig. 3**).

Key history findings include[3]:

- Medications, such as chemotherapy agents, are a known cause of arresting nail matrix.
- Illness, including pneumonia, malaria, leprosy, may also cause these lines.
- Poisoning, such as arsenic, thallium, and carbon monoxide, have traditionally been associated with this finding.
- Other conditions, such as childbirth, myocardial infarction, heart failure, renal failure, psoriasis, and sickle cell anemia, may also cause these lines.

Physical examination findings:

- Transverse, nonblanchable white bands that parallel and follow the contour of the lunula may be found.[4]
- Similar to Beau lines, providers should measure the distance from proximal nail fold to determine the time of insult to the nail matrix.

The differential diagnosis of Mees lines includes Muehrcke lines, Beau lines, and leukonychia punctate. Leukonychia punctate is the most common type of leukonychia and is typically caused by minor trauma.[3] There is no routine laboratory workup unless potential toxic exposure is suspected. A heavy metal workup is indicated in those patients. As with Beau lines, patients presenting with Mees lines should be reassured that this nail abnormality will disappear as the nail grows out unless there is repeated insults from the underlying systemic disorder or medication.

Terry Nails

First described by Richard Terry, a British physician, in 1954 when he noticed approximately 80 of 100 patients with cirrhosis of the liver presented with reddish, moon-shaped discoloration of their nails. The nail discoloration is thought to be associated with distal telangiectasias.[6] Terry nails have been linked to hepatic failure, heart failure, type 2 diabetes mellitus, and as part of the normal aging process.[6] Patients typically present with nonpainful, reddish/brown bands at the distal edge of the free nail, absence of the lunula, and white discoloration of most of the nail plate. All fingernails are usually affected (**Fig. 4**).

Key history findings include:

- Alcohol consumption as Terry nails is historically linked to hepatic cirrhosis from chronic alcohol use.[6]

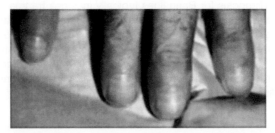

Fig. 3. Mees lines. (*From* Talley NJ, O'Connor S. Clinical examination: a systematic guide to physical diagnosis. 6th edition. Sydney (Australia): Elsevier. 2010; with permission.)

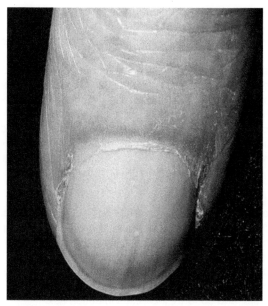

Fig. 4. Terry lines. (*From* James WD, Elston DM, Berger TG, et al. Andrews' diseases of the skin: clinical dermatology. 11th edition. London: Saunders/Elsevier; 2011. p. 741–82; with permission.)

- Comorbid medical conditions, such cardiac failure, type 2 diabetes mellitus, hyperthyroidism, and renal failure, have also been associated with this finding.

Physical examination findings:
- Inspection of all 10 fingernails typically shows a 0.5- to 3.0-mm-wide reddish/brown transverse band at the distal edge of the free nail with whitish discoloration of the remainder of nail plate with disappearance of the lunula.[6]
- The age of patients is important in determining the cause of this nail finding. Although this sign can be a normal part of the aging process, discovery of this finding in a younger person should trigger further workup.

The differential diagnosis of Terry nails includes Lindsay nails and Mees lines. Laboratory workup should be dictated by full physical examination of patients and evaluation for any underlying systemic illnesses that may have contributed to the development of this nail abnormality. Liver function tests, renal function evaluation, thyroid-stimulating hormone, and hemoglobin A1c may be part of the workup for this nonspecific nail finding. There is no specific treatment of Terry nails other than treatment of any underlying hepatic, cardiac, or renal disorders and patient reassurance.

Fingernail Onychomycosis

Onychomycosis is the term used to describe a fungal infection of the nail. It affects approximately 4% of the population in the United States and Europe[7] and represents a quarter to half of all onychopathies.[8] Fingernail onychomycosis is most common in women and in persons between the third and fourth decade of life because of repeated work-related injuries.[9] These infections are typically caused by *Trichophyton* sp (specifically *Trichophyton rubrum*), *Microsporum*, or *Epidermophyton*.

Occasionally, nondermatophyte molds and yeasts can also cause onychomycosis.[7] Risk factors for contracting fingernail onychomycosis include damage to the nail, history of diabetes mellitus, increasing age, genetic factors, occupational exposure to chemicals or wet environments, increased physical activity, climate, and frequency of travel.[7] Complications associated with untreated fingernail onychomycosis include cellulitis, chronic paronychia, impaired or lost tactile function, and possible infection of others.[7] Onychomycosis is classified into 5 main clinical types: distal subungual, proximal subungual, white superficial, total dystrophic, and candida onycomycosis.[4] Fingernail onychomycosis may present unilaterally, with single or multiple nails involved, and typically associated with concomitant tinea corporis or tinea capitis.[7] Patients may complain of pain, discomfort, brittleness, lack of nail growth, onycholysis, or unpleasant aesthetic appearance of their nails.

Key history findings include:
- Comorbid health conditions are important to notate, as diabetes mellitus (an independent risk factor for the development of onychomycosis), psoriasis, human immunodeficiency virus/AIDS, and other immunosuppressed conditions increase the risk of development of onychomycosis.[7]
- Work-related activity that results in trauma to the nail (ie, typing, athletes) or wet work environments (ie, landscapers, hairdressers, restaurant work, housewives, daycare workers, and so forth) increases infection risk.
- There is an increased risk with frequent travel to hot, humid climates.
- Habits, such nail biting and cuticle manipulation, cause disruption of normal barriers to infection.
- Hobbies, such as gardening, swimming, and so forth, increase the infection risk.
- Nail care habits, such as the use of manicurists, increase infection risk because of manipulation and instrumentation.
- Other skin conditions include tinea capitis or tinea corporis.

Physical examination findings:
- Distal subungual onychomycosis is the most common finding and typically coincides with tinea pedis. The nail will have hyperkeratosis of the distal nail plate and bed with or without onycholysis and may have a yellowish or whitish discoloration of the nail that becomes more pronounced as the infection continues.[4]
- Proximal subungual onychomycosis presents with a normal nail plate early in the infection but progresses to leukonychia of the proximal nail. The infection begins when the dermatophyte penetrates the proximal nail fold area.[4]
- White superficial onychomycosis is rare in fingernails and presents with white, crumbling lesions on the surface of the nail plate. This condition is more often seen in children than adults and is typically due to *Trichophyton mentagrophytes*.[7]
- Total dystrophic onychomycosis may begin as any of the other types of onychomycosis that then progresses to involve the entire nail. Patients will present with thickened nails with subungual hyperkeratosis and eventually total destruction of the nail plate.[7]
- Candida onychomycosis typically presents similar to distal and lateral subungual onychomycosis, and paronychia often coincides with the nail plate findings.[7]

The differential diagnosis for onychomycosis includes nail psoriasis, lichen planus, trauma, eczema, yellow nail syndrome, and nail changes due to normal aging.[7] Multiple KOH stains and or fungal cultures should be performed before completely ruling out onychomycosis, as it may be difficult to isolate fungal organisms or hyphal elements with just one attempt.[4] Areas to obtain nail elements for KOH or fungal culture for each type of onychomycosis are as follows:

- Distal subungual onychomycosis: Use a curette or nail elevator to obtain subungual debris or send nail clipping.[4]
- Proximal subungual onychomycosis: A curette or scalpel blade may be needed to obtain debris from the proximal nail bed.[4]
- White superficial onychomycosis: Use a scalpel blade to scrape the surface of the white, crumbling area.[7]
- Total dystrophic onychomycosis: Obtain subungual debris or nail bed clipping.[4]
- Candida onychomycosis: Obtain debris from the proximal and lateral edges as well as under the nail.[7]

To date there is no one ideal treatment of onychomycosis, and current therapeutic agents typically result in around a 30% mycological cure rate with optimal treatment.[7] Oral agents are generally more effective than topical agents, although newer topical agents have shown promise.[8] According to the British Association of Dermatologists, topical treatments should be used if there is limited involvement of the nail plate (ie, lack of matrix involvement, less than 3 nails affected, early distal and superficial white onychomycosis), if systemic agents are contraindicated, or in combination with oral agents.[7,8]

Other considerations in selecting therapy include the age of patients, comorbid health conditions, cost, compliance, drug-drug interactions, and possible adverse effects.[7] The two oral agents used as the first-line treatment of onychomycosis are itraconazole and terbinafine. Both require 6 weeks of treatment of fingernail onychomycosis, liver function test, and complete blood counts before treatment and are contraindicated in chronic or active liver disease. Terbinafine has fewer drug-drug interactions and has been shown to be superior for the treatment of dermatophyte infections than itraconazole.[7] Topical agents include amorolfine 5% lacquer, ciclopirox 8% lacquer, and efinaconazole 10% solution.[7] Patients should be monitored for improvement in nail appearance, mycological cure rates, and development of complications, such as paronychia.

Onycholysis

Onycholysis is the term used to describe the distal separation of the nail plate from the underlying nail bed. It is a nonspecific nail finding and is the third most common nail disorder seen in practice. (Cashman) Onycholysis is associated with many systemic disorders but is more commonly secondary to trauma or irritant or allergic contact dermatitis.[1] Patients typically present with white discoloration of the nail plate. Tenderness or fragility of nail plate may occur on manipulation (**Fig. 5**).

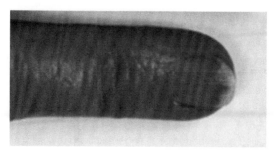

Fig. 5. Onycholysis.

Key history findings include:
- Occupations such as wet work environments (ie, bartenders, housewives, and so forth).
- Comorbid conditions such as nutritional deficiencies, hyperthyroidism or hypothyroidism, pregnancy, chemotherapy agents are associated causes of onycholysis.[3]
- Trauma from housework, manicures and other industrial work may be noted.
- Coexistent dermatologic conditions including verruca vulgaris, psoriasis, onychomycosis, and lichen planus can lead to.

Physical examination findings:
- There is usually no sign of inflammation and a normal appearing nail plate.
- There is distal separation of the nail plate from the nail bed with white discoloration of the nail plate.
- There is splinter hemorrhages if due to trauma.
- The number of nails involved correlates with the underlying cause. Hyperthyroidism can cause brown discoloration with onycholysis of most nails. This condition is termed *Plummer nails*.[10]
- Discoloration of the nail plate may result from secondary contamination of *Pseudomonas* or *Candida* sp of the open space formed when the nail plate separated from the nail bed.[3]

The differential diagnosis of onycholysis includes Lindsay nails, Plummer nails, onychomycosis, psoriasis, and lichen planus. Although there is no routine laboratory workup for onycholysis, a KOH may be performed to rule out onychomycosis. Treatment should be aimed at reassuring patients that the condition is benign, proper nail care techniques, and treatment of any secondary infection or underlying systemic or dermatologic disorder.

Longitudinal Melanonychia

Longitudinal melanonychia (LM) is often a difficult patient encounter in dermatology. The cause of this nail finding can range from benign to malignant and is often difficult to diagnosis on visual inspection. The most common causes of LM involving multiple nails include racial factors, trauma, and other systemic factors, such as inherited diseases, pregnancy, drug induced, and endocrine and rheumatologic disorders.[11,12] Approximately 80% of African American and 50% of Hispanic persons can develop these lines with the aging process.[11] LM associated with a single nail can be due to various inflammatory nail disorders, benign or malignant nail tumors, nail matrix nevus, and nail matrix melanoma.[11] Patients typically present with nonpainful, linear pigmentation that extends the length of the nail (**Fig. 6**).

Key history findings include:
- Recent trauma to help rule out hematoma formation.
- Comorbid conditions as LM may be caused by certain endocrine and rheumatologic conditions.
- Length of time pigmentation has been present to determine if pigmentation is acute or chronic in nature.
- Current hobbies to rule out the possibility of microtrauma.
- Nail care habits to identify potential causes of the pigmentation.

Physical examination[12]:
- Perform a detailed examination of all fingernails and toenails, proximal and lateral nail folds, and oral mucosa.

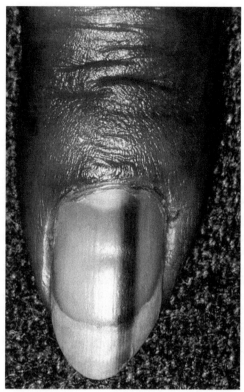

Fig. 6. LM. (*From* James WD, Elston DM, Berger TG, et al. Andrews' diseases of the skin: clinical dermatology. 11th edition. London: Saunders/Elsevier; 2011. p. 741–82; with permission.)

- Be sure to document single nail or multiple nail involvement.
- Measure the width of pigmentation and detail overall pigmentation pattern (homogeneous or heterogeneous appearance).

Dermoscopy with immersion medium is a noninvasive method to narrow the differential diagnosis of LM.[12] Despite the advances of dermoscopy, histopathology remains the gold standard for evaluation of LM. Biopsy for histopathologic examination should be performed if the origin of LM cannot be determined and/or patients meet the A, B, or E criteria (A = age, B = brown to black band of 3 mm or more breadth, E = extension of pigment to proximal and/or lateral nail fold) as this is highly suspicious for nail melanoma.[11] Treatment of LM ranges from reassurance to surgical interventions. A carefully elicited history and detailed physical examination are crucial for determining the cause of LM.

Subungual Hematoma

Subungual hematoma is the most common cause of brown-black nail pigmentation. It may present as LM and requires a detailed history and physical examination. It is the result of trauma to the nail unit that patients may or may not be aware of. Patients typically present with reddish-black to brown-black pigmentation under the nail. It is often alarming to patients because of the long length of time blood accumulation can remain in the subungual space. The pigmentation may be present on a single nail or multiple depending on the traumatic event. These lesions are typically nonpainful unless caused by an acute traumatic event (**Fig. 7**).

Key history findings include:
- Recent trauma to the nail.
- Current hobbies as repetitive microtrauma from shoes often unnoticed by patients
- Timing to determine the chronicity of the discoloration.

Physical examination findings include:
- Perform a detailed examination of all fingernails and toenails, proximal and lateral nail folds, and oral mucosa.
- It typically involves a single nail.
- There are round or linear bands of reddish-black or brown-black pigmentation.
- Pigmentation will progress distally with nail plate growth.

The differential diagnosis of subungual hematoma is large and includes racial longitudinal melanonychia, onychomycosis, nevi of the nail matrix, drug-induced longitudinal melanonychia, and melanoma of the nail matrix.[12] Dermoscopy of the lesions should be performed when possible and will show homogeneous pigmentation color, globular pattern, and peripheral fading.[11] A biopsy may be necessary if the subungual hematoma does not progress distally, as this occurrence has been associated with neovascularization due to a tumor under the nail plate.[12] Treatment of subungual hematoma consists of reassurance of patients if the diagnosis is certain and monitoring for progression of the pigmentation distally as the nail plate grows keeping in mind the rate of growth of the nail involved. A biopsy is indicated for any atypical features.

Melanoma of the Nail Matrix

Melanoma of the nail matrix may also present as a type of LM. Patients typically present with a brown to black band of pigmentation on only one nail. It is nonpainful and

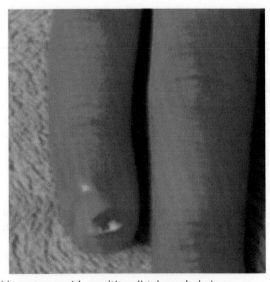

Fig. 7. Subungual hematoma with resulting distal onycholysis.

does not disappear as the nail grows out. Melanoma of the nail matrix usually occurs in individuals aged 50 to 70 years and will have no clinical or historical findings to suggest its occurrence (**Fig. 8**).

Key history findings are the same as for LM and include:
- Trauma
- Comorbid conditions
- Length of time pigmentation present: new pigmentation in older persons highly suspicious for nail melanoma
- Hobbies: used to eliminate traumatic causes
- Nail care habits
- Family history of melanoma

Physical examination findings include:
- LM of one nail
- Breadth of pigmentation typically greater than 3 mm
- +/- Hutchinson sign: nail bed, matrix, and nail plate pigment that extends to the proximal and/or lateral nail folds[11]

Dermoscopy should be used initially, if possible, to evaluate for brown background, irregular margins, and noncontinuous, nonparallel lines.[11] Unfortunately dermoscopy is not useful in thick nails or if the pigmentation is completely black.[11] Histopathologic examination is required for the evaluation of suspected nail matrix melanoma. If performed properly, it will not cause permanent nail dystrophy and must be used in clinically or historically unexplained single-nail pigmented bands.[11] Treatment of melanoma of the nail matrix is surgical. Surgical excision ranges from removal of the entire nail apparatus to amputation of the affected digit depending on the type of melanoma discovered, digit involved (thumbs are essential for grasping), and aesthetic outcomes.[12] After treatment, patients and first-degree relatives should continue monthly self-skin examinations and routine full-body skin examinations with their dermatology provider.

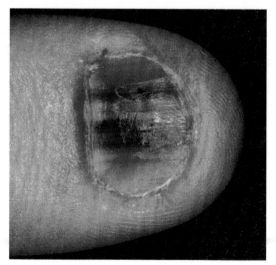

Fig. 8. Nail melanoma. (*From* Swartz MH. The skin: in textbook of physical diagnosis. 6th edition. Philadelphia: Elsevier; 2009. p. 137–95; with permission.)

Table 1 Selected nail patterns		
Pitting	Small pinpoint depressions in the nail plate	Psoriasis, eczema, lichen planus, alopecia areata
Leukonychia punctate	Linear white lines in the nail plate	Minor trauma
Onycholysis	White discoloration of the nail plate in area nonadhered to nail bed Discoloration may occur with secondary infection in the open space	Psoriasis, trauma, contact dermatitis, thyroid disease
Beau lines	Transverse furrows or grooves	Infection, medications, trauma, systemic and cutaneous disease
Mees lines	Transverse, nonblanchable white bands	Arsenic, thallium, or carbon monoxide poisoning; heart failure; childbirth; infection; chemotherapy agents; renal failure
Muehrcke lines	Multiple transverse white lines that blanch and do not grow out with nail plate	Hypoalbuminemia, chemotherapy agents
Lindsay nails	Half and half nails: half pink, half white	Renal failure
Terry nails	Narrow reddish/brown transverse band distally with white coloration of most of nail	Hepatic failure, heart failure, type 2 diabetes mellitus, normal aging
LM	Pigmented linear discoloration that may extend the length of the nail	Drug induced, endocrine disorders, genetic, racial, nevi of nail matrix, melanoma of nail matrix

Data from Refs.[3,5,10]

SUMMARY

Nail disorders account for around 10% of all dermatologic conditions and may provide an initial sign of systemic disease. Although many nail signs are nonspecific, recognition of these findings along with a detailed history and physical examination can guide providers to the proper diagnosis (**Table 1**).

REFERENCES

1. Cashman MW, Sloan SB. Nutrition and nail disease. Clin Dermatol 2010;28(4): 420–5.

2. Singh G, Haneef NS. Nail changes and disorders among the elderly. Indian J Dermatol Venereol Leprol 2005;71(6):386–92.

3. Zaiac MN, Daniel CR. Nails in systemic disease. Dermatol Ther 2002;15:99–106.

4. Daniel CR. Diagnosis of onychomycosis and other nail disorders: a pictorial atlas. New York: Springer-Verlag New York; 1996.

5. Avery H, Cooper HL, Karim A. Unilateral Beau's lines associated with a fractured olecranon. Australas J Dermatol 2010;51:145–6.

6. Nia AM, Ederer S, Dahlem KM, et al. Terry's nails: a window to systemic diseases. AM J Med 2011;124(7):602–4.

7. Eisman S, Sinclair R. Fungal nail infection: diagnosis and management. BMJ 2014;348:g1800.
8. Taheri A, Davis SA, Huang KE, et al. Onychomycosis treatment in the United States. Cutis 2015;95:15–21.
9. Gelotar P, Vachhani S, Patel B, et al. The prevalence of fungi in fingernail onychomycosis. J Clin Diagn Res 2013;7(2):250–2.
10. Fawcett RS, Linford S, Stulberg DL. Nail abnormalities: clues to systemic disease. Am Fam Physician 2004;69(6):1417–24.
11. Piraccini BM, Dika E, Fanti PA. Tips for diagnosis and treatment of nail pigmentation with practical algorithm. Dermatol Clin 2015;33:185–95.
12. Braun RP, Baran R, Le Gal FA, et al. Diagnosis and management of nail pigmentations. J Am Acad Dermatol 2007;56(5):835–47.

Moving?

Make sure your subscription moves with you!

To notify us of your new address, find your **Clinics Account Number** (located on your mailing label above your name), and contact customer service at:

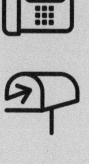

Email: journalscustomerservice-usa@elsevier.com

800-654-2452 (subscribers in the U.S. & Canada)
314-447-8871 (subscribers outside of the U.S. & Canada)

Fax number: 314-447-8029

Elsevier Health Sciences Division
Subscription Customer Service
3251 Riverport Lane
Maryland Heights, MO 63043

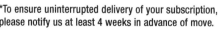

Did you know you could earn
15 AMA Category 1 CME credits
by reading this issue?

Physician Assistant Clinics subscribers can access online CME tests based on each issue to **earn up to 60 AMA Category 1 CME credits per year** (15 credits per issue, 4 issues per year).

If you are a current subscriber, visit **physicianassistant.theclinics.com/CME** to claim access and to begin taking the exams.

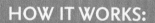
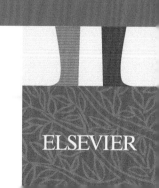

Printed and bound by CPI Group (UK) Ltd, Croydon, CR0 4YY

03/10/2024

01040392-0015